MOTIVATING PEOPLE

PRACTICAL STRATEGIES AND TECHNIQUES FOR SUPPORT WORKERS

ROBIN DYNES

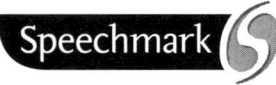

First published in 2014 by
Speechmark Publishing Ltd
St Mark's House, Shepherdess Walk, London N1 7BQ, United Kingdom
www.speechmark.net

002-5875 Printed in the United Kingdom by CMP (uk) Limited.

British Library Cataloguing in Publication Data
A catalogue record for this book is available from the British Library.

ISBN: 978 0 86388 958 5

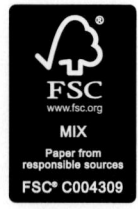

CONTENTS

INTRODUCTION

Motivating service users is one of the biggest challenges facing staff working in all types of support roles. Miller and Rollnick (1991, p19) tell us that 'it is no longer sensible to blame a client for being unmotivated to change ... Motivation is an inherent and central part of the professional's task'. A service user may lack motivation to accept help, socialise, change unacceptable behaviour, take medication or follow a more healthy lifestyle. They may be resistant, deny any need to change or sabotage attempts to help them. These are the kinds of situations faced by front-line staff on a daily basis.

Who this book is for

This book is aimed at all types of support workers, healthcare assistants, social workers, occupational therapists, youth workers, employment officers, tutors, counsellors, coaches and managers. In fact, it will be useful to staff working across a wide variety of environments, such as residential homes, day centres and education, as well as nursing and probation. Many of the front-line staff working in these environments have limited opportunities to go on courses to learn techniques which will support them in their day-to-day work motivating service users to participate in activities, arousing their interest in making changes or altering unacceptable behaviour.

What is offered?

This book provides some ideas, strategies and techniques which can be integrated into day-to-day work. Although drawn from a number of approaches, which include motivational interviewing, cognitive behaviour therapy, solution-focused therapy and neuro-linguistic programming, among others, you do not need to be a qualified counsellor, social worker, nurse or therapist to use them. In fact, you can use them with your children, partner, parents, colleagues and friends. They are strategies which I have used over the past 30 years working in the

Probation Service, the National Health Service and Social Services, and in adult education to support students.

The book is divided into two parts:

Part 1 contains some general information about the process of change and on using the strategies and techniques discussed in Part 2.

Part 2 provides a range of strategies, approaches and suggestions which can be incorporated into daily practice.

As it is envisaged that the book will be utilised in a wide range of settings, the terms 'service user' and 'person' have been used throughout to indicate the person with whom you are working. Feel free to change the terminology, however – to 'patient', 'client', 'student', 'resident', and so on – to suit your own situation. Likewise, the term 'support worker' can be replaced with the title of your role, be that healthcare assistant, nurse, mentor, tutor or youth worker.

How to use this book

Start by reading through Part 1 and scanning through the rest of the book to get an overall picture of what is provided. The suggestions offered are not intended to replace professional training in the various therapeutic approaches – attending appropriate courses is advised – but take from them ideas which can be put into practice and used by all staff, including receptionists and volunteers.

There are many ways in which additional knowledge can be gained, and the basic ideas presented here can be built on and incorporated into daily work routines. A motivational group can be formed to discuss issues and improve practice. One member of staff might like to take on the role of a 'motivational champion' and organise meetings. Discussions can be held on particular techniques, and role plays invented to practise them. After using a strategy with a service user, the experience can be reviewed and suggestions given to improve skill. This can be particularly useful when considering how language is used and sentences are framed. Every encounter with service users is different and this is an area in which practitioners can always find ways to improve. It may also be possible to record some role plays to aid feedback.

These types of learning forums provide essential ongoing coaching and skill maintenance. Time and practice are needed – usually a few months – for individuals to build up confidence and comfort in using new approaches.

Further reading in the various therapeutic approaches will enhance your knowledge. As well as distance-learning courses, there are now many videos available for training purposes. While it is unlikely that all members of staff could attend a wide range of courses in different therapeutic disciplines – many short introductory training sessions are available in most – individuals could attend particular courses and then cascade their learning and give feedback on practice to others. You may have a member of staff who has been trained, or is able to involve someone who has expertise in a particular approach, to give individual or group supervision or provide short training sessions.

These are just some suggestions for how the strategies and approaches in this book can be built on to improve staff ability to motivate and support service users.

Built-in flexibility

The book has been structured to provide maximum flexibility. When generally aiming to work in a way that motivates service users, it can be dipped into for ideas. In addition, it suggests approaches that can be used when someone:

- acknowledges there is a concern and wants help with it
- has started to make changes and wants support to help them maintain those
- accepts there is an issue, but thinks it is someone's else's job to fix it
- denies that there is a problem and is unwilling to do anything about it.

It will also help staff build on existing skills and learn new techniques.

PART 1

UNDERSTANDING HOW SELF-MOTIVATION IS DEVELOPED

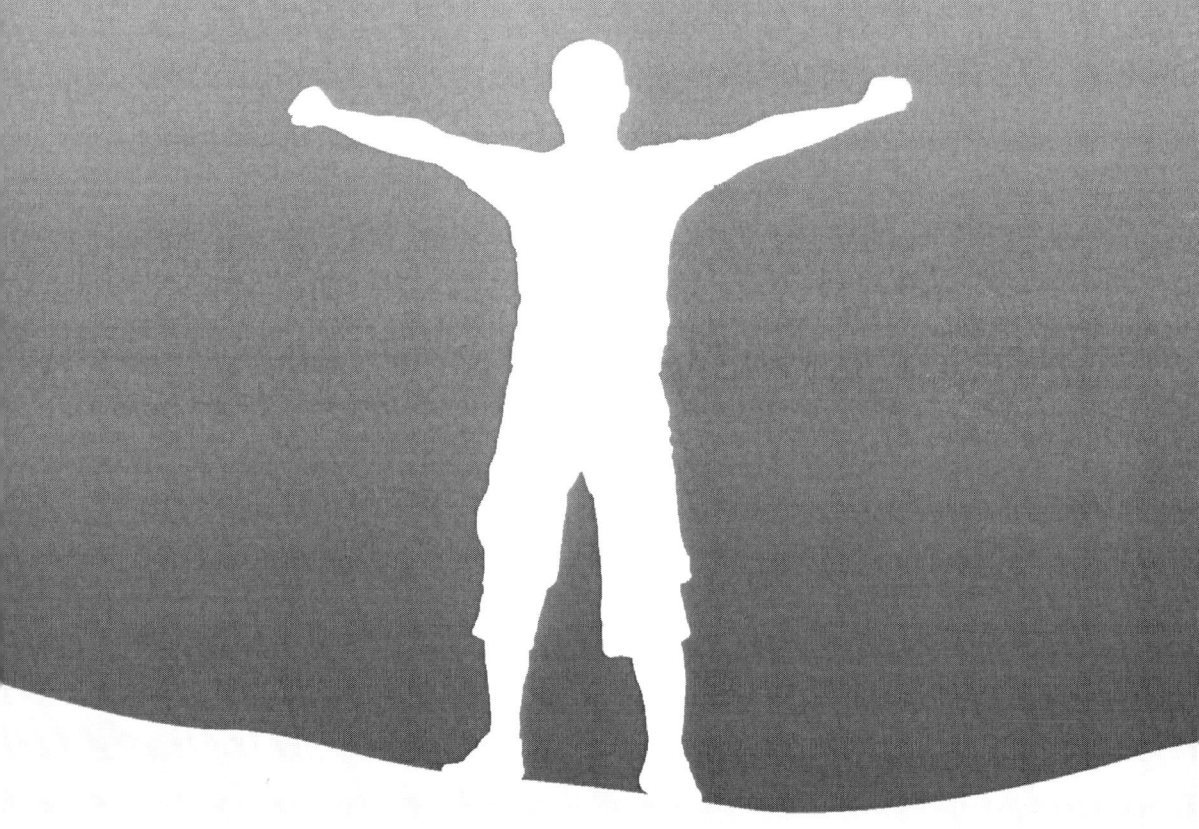

Striving to motivate others

A strong desire to help others, combined with a lack of motivation in service users, can result in feelings of inadequacy, failure, frustration and stress. It can also lead us to think it is our fault when someone resists taking action to deal with their situation. There are many things which influence an individual's lack of motivation to take action. These vary from internal thoughts and fears to external influences, such as particular circumstances and unpredictable events, on top of which we have only limited contact time with each service user – anything from a few minutes to a few hours each day depending on the setting. For some, contact may be once a week or less. Service users' resistance to change is not personal to us as workers and we should not allow it to become so.

It is very easy, especially for new recruits to a service, to get sucked into taking on service users' personal problems and to try to fight their internal conflicts for them. Allowing the struggle to become personal in this way will, undoubtedly, be followed by feelings of helplessness, inadequacy or failure in the worker. This can quite quickly lead to stress and to feeling that this type of work is not for them.

Some understanding about motivation and some strategies and techniques to help individuals become self-motivated when they become 'stuck' or are resistant to change are essential, both in controlling stress experienced by staff and for empowering service users.

Becoming stuck in a motivational bog

Service users are frequently stuck in a motivational 'bog' or 'quicksand' that threatens to engulf them. They appear to be paralysed and unable to decide what to do or, indeed, unable to muster up the enthusiasm or energy to take action or adapt to necessary changes.

They may not recognise that they need to take action to change their situation. This may be because they wilfully ignore aspects of their circumstances, do not see the need, or fear the consequences of making

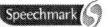

any changes, or do not have the skills or confidence to be able to achieve different outcomes successfully. So they stick with what they feel is safe.

There may be aspects of their behaviour or attitudes which are not acceptable to others in the community or environment in which they live. These may have become ingrained over a long period of time, or may even have been established within their family culture over several generations.

Working with people who lack motivation or do not see the need for change can become draining for staff, resulting in burn-out and lack of job satisfaction, unless they adopt methods beyond those commonly used to motivate service users.

Some methods commonly used to motivate individuals

Some of the most common approaches used to motivate service users are given below. These work on some occasions, but are less effective at other times or with people who lack motivation and are reluctant to reach a decision about their situation or take any action (indeed, some may lack awareness or be wilfully ignoring that there is a problem).

The enthusiastic worker

This is the lively and eager worker who 'jollies' everyone along. This person outlines all the benefits of doing something and enthusiastically cajoles service users into taking part. Sometimes this does not work well: the service user may feel patronised and resentful while appearing to comply. It can also be difficult for the worker to keep up this level of 'jolliness' – making it exhausting for both worker and service user alike.

Making frequent but brief contacts

This can work well with many of those service users who are new to day centres or residential homes. Too much contact and socialising can be overwhelming, particularly if the person has been isolated, has poor socialising skills or lacks confidence. A very brief word or a smile as you catch their gaze from time to time can start to create trust, build

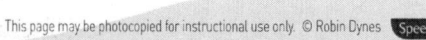

confidence and draw them into longer conversations and into taking part in activities. However, this can be less effective with someone who resents being in the centre or home or has long-established maladaptive behaviour or other issues.

Doing the logical thing

It may seem logical that particular services or activities are valuable to the service user. These are explained and offered. After some discussion of what is available, agreement is reached that it would be beneficial for the person to take part in them. The individual is then expected to be motivated to take part in what has been decided. This common approach can work well as long as the person wants to collaborate and what is provided will meet their needs.

Asking the person to help you

This might be to help you with laying tables, watering plants, giving advice about something or preparing a room for an activity, among other things. You do need to make sure that you actually require help, however, otherwise this can come across as patronising. Also, you need to make sure that what you are requesting is within the person's abilities.

Adopting a 'caring' role

In this instance it is assumed that if you care for and nurture the service user, this will ultimately lead to them wanting to engage in the services offered. This type of unconditional one-direction giving can be draining and can result in the worker feeling worn out. The service user, in turn, will probably still feel stuck and unmotivated.

Minimising 'involvement' or what is 'required'

People often fear new experiences because they do not know what will be expected of them. They fear not being able to do what is required, or looking stupid. To try to involve these people in activities, creating a situation in which they can be an observer or have a minor role may be enough to help them decide whether or not to participate. This enables them to acclimatise themselves to the situation and feel more confident about their ability to cope with it before becoming fully involved. It can

 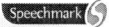

work well with people who have some motivation but lack confidence – it is less effective with someone who is not motivated.

Adopting a 'minimum responsibility' attitude

Services are provided and it is the service user's responsibility to cooperate and show some willingness to participate. They may be invited to arranged activities, but if they show a lack of motivation, the worker regards them as not being at a stage when they are ready to take part, as being depressed, as having decided the activities are not for them, or that there are other factors beyond the worker's control. In this situation, individuals who lack motivation are often left to their own devices until a time when they might become cooperative.

Introducing people to something with which they are familiar

The service user may have a particular talent for doing something. This may be for drawing, writing poetry or doing a particular craft, such as embroidery or playing the piano. The person is more likely to participate in activities in areas in which they feel confident or can share their special talent or wisdom. It reinforces their self-esteem and provides a motivator for being involved.

Strengths and limitations of these methods

These and similar types of approach are useful in different situations, usually with service users who are already motivated in some way. The strengths of these methods include instilling hope in the service user, provided that the worker believes the service user can achieve their goal or participate in the activities suggested; giving the service user a 'kick start'; offering a positive attitude; helping, in some instances, to establish some empathy; and the fact that they can be empowering.

However, for a large number of service users these methods do not meet their need as the methods often fail to:

- recognise the obstacles which have to be overcome or whether the person is able to make the change required

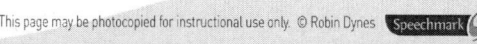

- take into account the price the person has to pay to make the change – often the fear of what will be lost is too high

- encourage self-responsibility

- acknowledge that what the worker sees as a benefit or as quite rational may not be seen as a benefit or rational by the service user

- recognise low self-esteem in a service user

- individualise the approach to the person concerned

- detect that what is seen as a negative consequence by the worker is not necessarily seen as negative by the service user.

In addition, such methods may:

- be seen as patronising by some

- result in service users complying, but feeling that they are being forced into doing something

- in some instances be difficult to maintain and result in staff feeling drained and exhausted

- result in people feeling dependent

- create problems with boundaries, such as ignoring or neglecting the needs of service users because they do not appear to be cooperative

- be vague about outcomes

- appear to be collaborative, but frequently are not.

Other approaches need to be applied that inspire self-motivation and address such issues as low self-esteem, difficulty with overcoming obstacles, socially unacceptable behaviour, and social stigmatisation (which increases a person's sense of poor self-value and ability).

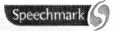

Confrontation versus self-motivation

The use of confrontational methods, such as threatening to withdraw a service and instructing or ordering someone to keep appointments or to do or not do something, rarely works in the long term. Self-motivation cannot be produced on command. It needs to be planted and cultivated within individuals. Make an effort to understand and focus on communication methods that create an environment in which individuals direct and control their own lives, and there will be fertile soil in which self-motivation can grow.

A process for developing self-motivation

Researchers James Prochaska and Carlo DiClemente (1982) developed an approach which showed the stages through which people pass during the process of change. These stages are as follows.

Pre-contemplation

The person may or may not be aware of the need for change and does not want to do anything about it. They may be unaware of the dangers or ignore the situation. The effort to make change may be too frightening or difficult and they do not see it as a possibility. The task at this stage is to raise awareness. (For the tactics to use, see Part 2, Section 1: 'Arousing interest'.)

Contemplation

The person knows or has become aware that there is a problem and, although undecided, is thinking about it. They may be pulled between 'do they' or 'don't they' do anything about it. The 'benefits' and 'losses' of doing something will be floating about in their head. During this stage you will need to reinforce movement in a positive direction. (For tactics, see Part 2, Section 2: 'Encouraging individuals to consider change'.)

Determination

There is a 'window' when the service user feels that change is possible and is open to developing ideas about how they can achieve it. This is the time to explore ideas, options and past skills which can be utilised, and new skills which can be developed, and to set goals and work out a plan. (For tactics, see Part 2, Section 3: 'Supporting people when they plan the change'.)

Action

This is the period during which the service user makes the changes. They may start by trying out one of the options. Lots of encouragement and support will be needed. (For tactics, see Part 2, Section 4: 'Guiding the person through planned actions'.)

Maintenance

Once changes have been made, the person will need to review plans and look at ways in which they can ensure the new behaviour is sustained. (For tactics, see Part 2, Section 5: 'Ensuring momentum is maintained'.)

Relapse

People often make several attempts to change a behaviour or habit before succeeding. This is especially true of behaviours which have been long standing, and relapses need to be anticipated and planned for. When a relapse occurs, the person may need to return to one of the previous stages. (For tactics, see Part 2, Section 6: 'Making positive use of relapses'.)

Permanent exit

Many professionals believe that the permanent resolution of a problem is not always possible; there is always a chance that, under pressure, it could return. (For tactics to avoid this, see Part 2, Section 7: 'Making sure change has been successfully achieved'.)

The techniques in Part 2 of this book have been arranged in a way that fits with the process of change discussed above. This does not mean that each tactic should be used only in the context of the heading under which it is placed. Many are transferable between sections and, indeed, should be used in that way as necessary. For example, using Strategy 7: 'Using

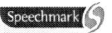

active listening skills' is imperative at all stages of the process, as is Strategy 20: 'Watching your language'.

Maslow's theory of motivation

It is essential always to keep in mind Maslow's 'hierarchy of needs', as shown in Figure 1.

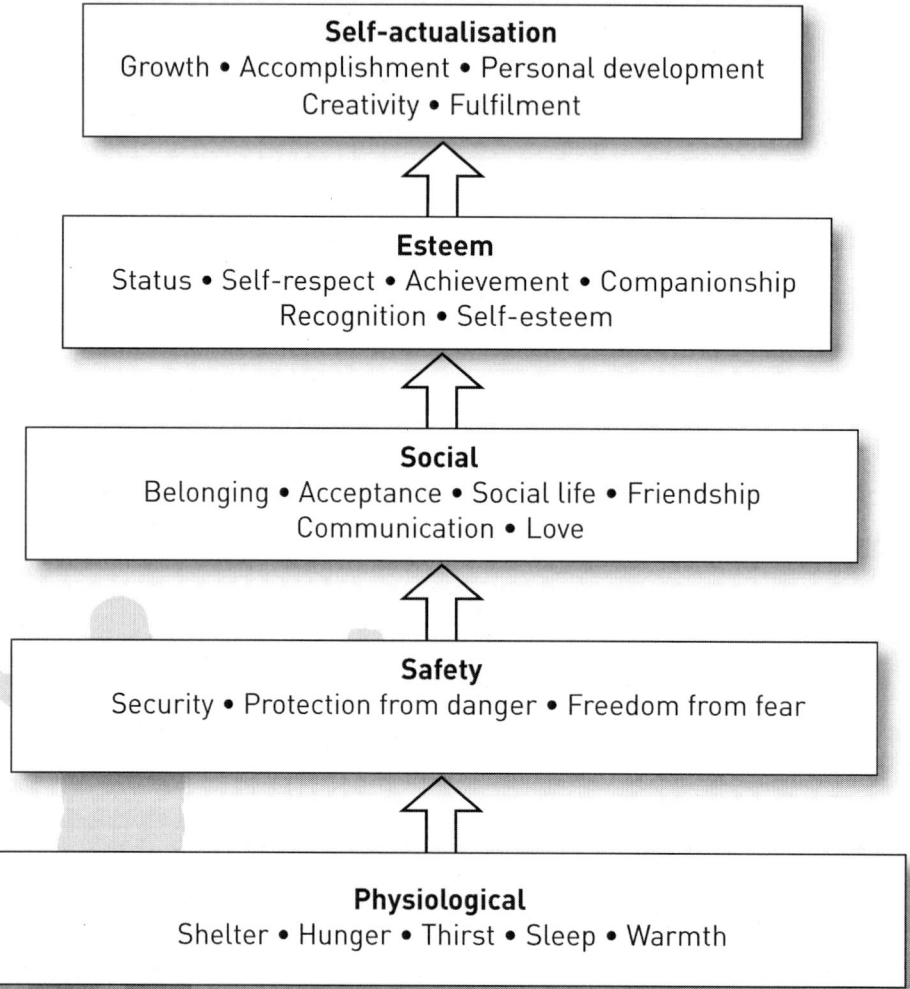

Self-actualisation
Growth • Accomplishment • Personal development
Creativity • Fulfilment

Esteem
Status • Self-respect • Achievement • Companionship
Recognition • Self-esteem

Social
Belonging • Acceptance • Social life • Friendship
Communication • Love

Safety
Security • Protection from danger • Freedom from fear

Physiological
Shelter • Hunger • Thirst • Sleep • Warmth

Figure 1 Maslow's hierarchy of needs

Figure 1 represents Maslow's original five-stage theory of motivation (Maslow, 1954). Later, he developed an eight-stage model (Maslow, 1971; Maslow & Lowery, 1999) which incorporated the following additional stages: 'cognitive', 'aesthetic' and 'transcendence'. Both models suggest that the lower levels of need must be satisfied before progressing to meet higher levels. Each person is able and has the desire to move up the hierarchy towards self-actualisation, although only a minority achieve this. The eight-stage model comprises:

1 **Physiological**: air, shelter, food, drink, sleep, etc. All the basic things the human body needs in order to function. If these needs are not met, we are likely to become ill.

2 **Safety**: protection from the elements and danger, security, order, law, etc. These provide a safe, orderly and predictable environment which is fair and in which we feel secure. Neglecting safety needs can result in severe stress and anxiety.

3 **Social**: belonging, acceptance, affection, friendship, love, relationships, etc. When 1 and 2 have been met, our needs become social and we seek acceptance, affection and love. Ignoring social needs can result in isolation, loneliness, depression and anxiety.

4 **Esteem**: self-respect, achievement, status, recognition, prestige, etc. Esteem needs are met when we feel comfortable and have gained status and success. Poor esteem can result in us feeling bad about ourselves, in a lack of confidence and in our failing to take risks to enable us to achieve.

5 **Cognitive**: knowledge, meaning, etc. We seek to gain an understanding of the world around us, to explore and want new experiences.

6 **Aesthetic**: appreciation of beautiful things, nature, art, music, etc. This provides a sense of oneness with nature.

7 **Self-actualisation**: realisation of personal potential; a sense of fulfilment is achieved. There is a feeling of harmony and of being connected.

8 **Transcendence**: we have a desire to help others self-actualise.

 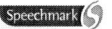

Most people consider that 'cognitive', 'aesthetic' and 'transcendence' are all aspects of 'self-actualisation' – Stage 5 in the original model. It is these features which are thought to create happiness. Failure to realise them can result in a feeling of emptiness or depression.

Maslow said that needs must be satisfied in the given order. However, this may not necessarily always be so, as most of us have deficiencies on different levels and only a small percentage of people achieve what he called 'self-actualisation'. Life is full of uncertainties – about health, employment, accidents and other unpredictable events, for example. Although individuals may have different tolerance levels for this and the stresses generated, we learn to live with them. Also, different cultures and backgrounds mean that many people have different values. Generally, in the West, we put higher value on lower-level needs, such as food, shelter, clothing, objects, status and achievements, than Eastern societies do. This influences what we see as basic needs. Consequently, many of us cope with deficiencies on most levels. Usually, the higher up the scale, the more deficiencies we may have. Consequently, it is helpful to let each individual guide you on what they see as their deficiencies and their basic need requirements. Whatever these needs are, the chances of change taking place and the person being able to successfully take steps towards self-actualisation are greater if they are met. (See Part 2, Strategy 2: 'Meeting basic needs'.)

Motivating people to change

In order for people to change, they need to be unhappy with their current situation in some way. This means they want:

- something they have not got

- to get away from something that feels uncomfortable

- to avoid unpleasant consequences.

For example, fear of loneliness may drive a person to want to make friends. Or wishing to gain status or provide a better standard of living for the family may motivate someone to study for qualifications.

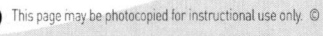 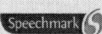

There may be a combination of reasons. However, having a reason to change is not a guarantee that someone *will* change as they may:

- not know how to make the changes

- feel they do not have the skills and the effort required is beyond them

- not feel dissatisfied enough to do anything about it

- be wilfully ignoring or unaware of the consequences of their behaviour (although you may be aware).

The importance of identifying stages in the change process

You may already be working with a service user and observe that they are unhappy with their situation. They may approach you and ask for help. You may be aware of someone doing something, but they are unaware or are ignoring the consequences. Alternatively, someone may be referred to you or brought to your attention by another member of staff. The initial task will be to identify the stage they are at in the change process. Having established that stage, appropriate strategies and techniques can then be used to move them on to the next stage.

This is very important as failure to motivate a service user may be due to a failure to identify the correct stage and use the most appropriate approach and style. So often, staff respond by identifying what needs to change or setting goals, whether or not the service user is ready, and try to jump straight into the action stage. This is the reason why so many fail to establish rapport and engage the service user. The person may appear to comply with what appear to be agreed actions, but then drops out at the first opportunity. These individuals can frequently come to be thought of as 'time wasters' or as being 'difficult'. Even if the service user wants to discuss a difficulty or change with you, they may only be at the contemplation stage and not yet ready for action.

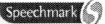

Speed of change

The speed with which individuals move from one stage of the process to another varies greatly. This will be influenced by both internal and external factors. There will be a for/against debate going on inside the service user's head and there may be a time limit and/or other external factors which mean that a decision has to be made or which adds enough weight to sway the argument. In a discussion, a service user may move from one stage to another in minutes; alternatively, they may be stuck in one stage for years, unable to weigh the decisional balance one way or another. This is particularly true in the 'contemplation', 'determination' and 'relapse' stages. Your task in the process is to enable them to shift the balance significantly in favour of taking action.

Self-management skills

Throughout the process of motivating someone, in this book the importance of the service user maintaining control is emphasised. It is easy to assume that this means the individual has the ability to self-manage their situation when, in fact, they need to learn some of the skills required to take control and do this effectively. Some self-management skills may be high on the agenda to enable the service user to carry out any actions required to make any planned changes or achieve their goals. This may entail you in teaching some of these skills. (See Part 2, Strategy 28: 'Sharing knowledge and teaching'.)

Ambivalence and relapse

Service users who are in a state of ambivalence about the need to change, who have relapsed or have changed their mind and are fluctuating back and forth – stuck in a decisional balance – should not be seen as hopeless or as failures. Ambivalence and relapse are part of the process of change and service users may relapse several times, learning from each experience, before finally achieving their goal. You will encounter both resistance and hesitancy. However, once the balance is weighed in favour of change, many things can suddenly seem possible and be achieved.

Using the strategies with groups

When using the strategies with groups, there are a few points to bear in mind. Some quiet people may fade into the background and others may become more dominant than usual. If discussing any personal issues, you will need to ensure that group members feel safe to do so. This will entail agreeing some ground rules to ensure that members respect each other and that everyone has the opportunity to express their opinions.

Some people may take extreme positions when discussing an issue, make inappropriate comments and try to tell others what they should do. Respond to these comments by reframing them (see Part 2, Strategy 18: 'Using reflective listening skills to roll with resistance') and emphasise each individual's personal control and choice.

Group members may also try to prove you wrong at times. Respond by asking participants what they think should be done. This allows solutions to come from them, rather than you being expected to provide answers. It also takes away any tensions brought about by anyone seeing you as an authoritative figure, and respects participants' own experience.

Some basic guiding principles

Below are some basic guiding principles which are helpful to keep in mind during the self-motivating process.

- Adopt an empathetic style and use active listening skills. This is essential throughout the process. The service user is the expert on themselves. Show positive regard and avoid any hint of being judgemental or critical. (See Part 2, Strategy 3: 'Showing positive regard' and Strategy 7: 'Using active listening skills'.)

- Take care with the language you use. This is important. Referring to something as a 'problem' can produce a defensive reaction. It is better to use language that is neutral and to substitute words such as

 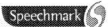

'concern' and 'issue'. (See Part 2, Strategy 20: 'Watching your language'.)

- Adopt a tone of providing information and informing the service user rather than trying to persuade them to change. If you drift into a tone of persuasion, you risk encountering resistance or the person becoming compliant but dropping out later.

- Identify the stage the person is at in the change process. Getting this wrong could mean moving on too quickly or applying the wrong techniques and failing to motivate the person.

- Be clear about the changes you believe the person needs to make. If you are not clear then any benefits explored will also appear vague and unpersuasive.

- Explore and clarify the risks of not making the change, as well as the advantages. Both will be needed to give weight to taking action. (See Part 2, Strategy 11: 'Using a motivational balance sheet'.)

- Identify and remove obstacles. This will include practical barriers, such as money, transport or lack of skills, as well as emotional or other intangible barriers, such as feeling anxious or lacking confidence.

- Confirm desire, ability, reason and need for, as well as commitment to, change before moving on to planning any actions. (See Part 2 Strategy 19: 'Prompting talk about change'.)

- Help the person clarify their goals, ensuring they take the lead. Make sure alternatives are explored so the person can make a choice. This helps increase their perception of being in control. (See Part 2, Strategy 23: 'Negotiating goals'.)

- Identify both 'driving' and 'restraining' forces that keep the person in a 'stuck' position. This will enable you to undermine and decrease forces which hinder movement and increase those which drive change. (See Part 2, Strategy 11: 'Using a motivational balance sheet'.)

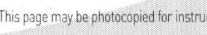 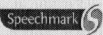

- Help the person break down their goals into small achievable steps and develop strategies to carry them out. This makes the goals seem possible and helps to build confidence in ability. (See Part 2, Strategy 24: 'Planning the change'.)

- Give clear and frequent feedback on progress. Use this to reinforce what the person is doing right and to enable them to learn from mistakes and generally build confidence. (See Part 2, Strategy 32: 'Monitoring progress'.)

- Use appropriate communication styles throughout the process – following, directing and guiding – as required. Move from one to the other as the situation demands. (See Part 2, Strategy 32: 'Monitoring progress'.)

These are also good principles to turn into questions to ask yourself when reflecting on how you are progressing with helping a service user become self-motivated. A questionnaire is provided in the Appendix.

Motivation and you

One of the biggest influences on motivation will be you. A sincere, genuine approach that puts the best interests of the service user at the centre of the task, whichever motivational techniques you choose to use, will have the greatest impact. It is also a fact that the opportunities are enormous for front-line workers in all environments to develop self-motivation in service users. This means that you are also in a position to produce the greatest positive effect on your service.

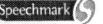

PART 2

STRATEGIES AND TECHNIQUES FOR MOTIVATING PEOPLE

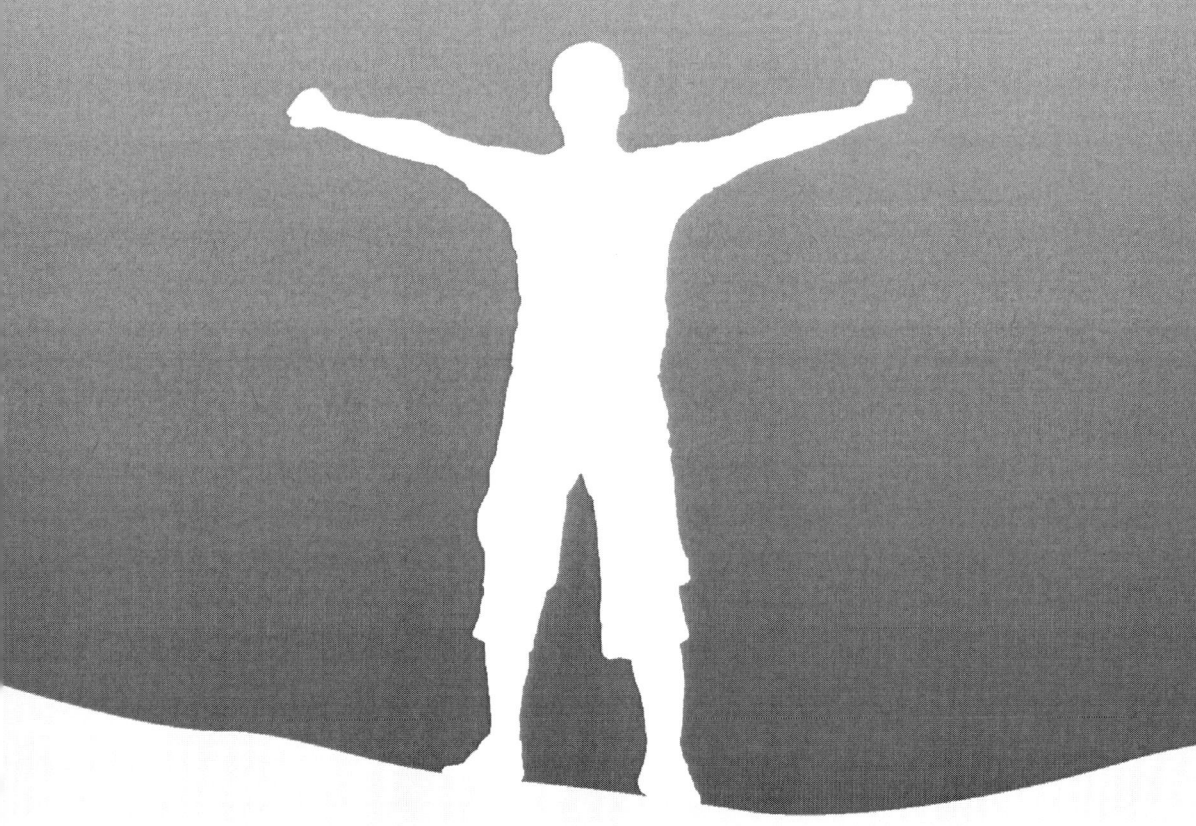

SECTION 1

Arousing interest (Pre-contemplation)

At this stage the person is unlikely to be considering the possibility of change or taking action. They may not see themselves as having a problem or they may blame other people for their predicament. They may deny the danger of the situation they are in or wilfully ignore what is obvious to others. They may have made several attempts to address the issue, failed, be demoralised and feel that trying to make any change is hopeless. Often, they may be withdrawn, uncommunicative and difficult to engage, or they may display behaviour that is disruptive to others. The problem may have become apparent to you as a tutor, group leader or carer. If you are a support or key worker, the person may have been referred to you to address the issues.

Your role at this stage is mainly to provide feedback and information to help raise awareness of the problem and the possibility of change. This includes raising doubts and increasing the person's perceptions of the risks and problems of continuing their current behaviour. Avoid using any 'scare tactics' because these may increase resistance as a result of the person's anxiety about their lack of ability to deal with their situation. It can also reinforce denial as a way of managing this.

The aim is to explore and enhance, in a matter-of-fact way, the person's understanding of the issue.

Strategy 1: Forming a contract

Introduction

Establishing rapport, active listening and showing positive regard are essential but are not adequate to allow you to carry out work with an individual. Integrity needs to be achieved through a contract that is understood and agreed by all parties involved. This incorporates a clear understanding of your authority, your purpose and the person's rights.

Depending on the setting in which you work, you may already have a relationship with the person. They may have been referred to you or have come to your attention because their behaviour has become a concern. They may not share your purpose or even acknowledge that there is a problem. You may be trying to generate motivation for a change that is thought to be more desirable or healthier for the person or the community in which they live. Integrity is maintained if the person understands the purpose of what you are doing.

How you could do this

It is likely that your setting already has guidelines for the work you do. However, you still need to make clear at the outset of meeting the person what you can expect of each other. Also, clarify any constraints, sanctions and resources that can be used. Bear in mind that your aim will be to work with the person to help them evaluate their situation and make a commitment to change. It remains their choice whether or not they decide to do so.

You need to be clear about any consequences if they decide either not to change or to make changes in a way that is unacceptable to your workplace or the law. Begin the process by using 'small talk' to establish some rapport and make the person feel at ease. This might be about the weather, how they got to the meeting, making sure they are seated comfortably, and so on. Next, clarify any necessary boundaries, such as time, limitation of authority and confidentiality.

If the person has been referred to you, or you have become aware that they have a problem, you might then move on to something like: *'What is your understanding of why we are meeting?'* If they have asked to meet with you, you might begin with *'What would you like to talk about today?'* This can then lead into exploration and clarification of the person's purpose. You can find this out by asking them a question such as: *'What would you like to gain from this chat/meeting?'*

You can then state your purpose: *'I would like to explore ...'* or *'Your tutor/group leader has informed me you have been upset and had to leave the class/group a few times. I understand you have been having a rough time recently and I wanted to see how things stand.'*

Generally, use open-ended questions that avoid *'Yes'* or *'No'* answers (for further explanation, see Strategy 7: 'Using active listening skills'). Maintain an attitude of curiosity and wanting to understand the behaviour or problem from the person's viewpoint. Find out about their values and beliefs (see Strategy 5: 'Establishing values and beliefs') and ask them how their behaviour or problem does or does not fit with those values. If it does not fit, they may acknowledge that change is needed. You can then ask them how they see this being resolved. They know themselves best and what works for them.

Phrase your questions along the lines of: *'What has helped you in the past in these circumstances?'* or *'What do you think would help resolve this?'* If you need to provide suggestions, pose them in a way that leaves the option of using them with the service user: *'What do you think about ...'*, *'Would it be helpful if ...?'* In this way the solutions are service user led and the person is far more likely to be motivated to work towards achieving them.

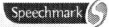

Comment

Highly confrontational approaches are likely to meet high resistance. It is more helpful to create an atmosphere in which the person can explore the issue openly and safely and come up with their own solutions. You will need to use open questions and reflections to check understanding of what has been agreed. Remember that the aim is to establish agreement about the work you are going to do together and to produce solution-focused statements that are self-motivating.

Strategy 2: Meeting basic needs

Introduction

Before anyone can begin contemplating making changes, either on their own or in a care or other setting, or having the motivation to take part in activities or learning, they need to feel both safe and that their basic needs are being met (see Maslow's hierarchy of needs in 'Maslow's theory of motivation' in Part 1). It is easy to assume in many settings that their needs *are* being met when in fact they are not. For example, the person may be homeless or under threat of eviction. They may live in a residential home but dislike, or have difficulty eating, the food available, or have problems sleeping ('Physiological' in Maslow's hierarchy). The person may have a fear of meeting people ('Social'), be worried about privacy or feel threatened ('Safety'). They may fear that working towards a qualification or making other changes, such as giving up drinking alcohol, will result in them losing friends ('Social') or their current status ('Esteem').

According to Maslow, we are motivated by our needs. The first four need levels – 'Physiological', 'Safety', 'Social' and 'Esteem' – are the essentials to help us function and cope with life. If there is a significant deficiency in one or more of these, it becomes extremely difficult to cope. For example, if a person does not feel sure that what they are going to say will remain confidential, they are unlikely to make disclosures (see Strategy 1: 'Forming a contract'), or if they are unhappy about the food, they may feel uncomfortable or refuse to take part in a party activity. A person working through marital problems or partnership break-up might not be able to focus their attention on an educational course. Deficiencies may also account for some aggressive or challenging behaviour – the person may not feel safe or that other needs are not being met. They may steal or behave in an unacceptable way to meet their perceived need. It may be essential to address self-esteem or other lower-level needs before the person feels able to make changes or to move on to achieve some growth and development.

How you could do this

Sometimes these deficiencies may be apparent or the person vocalises them and they can be addressed. At other times they may be disguised. The only indication may be seen through body language or the person being stressed, perhaps being reluctant to engage or isolating themselves. For example, a person may be upset and say they are lonely, but the underlying reason they avoid joining a class or group may be a fear of socialising ('Safety').

To discover the root cause you could say something like: *'You say that joining the coffee morning activity would help you get to know other people, but I can see from your expression that you are not totally comfortable with this. What is causing you to have doubts?'* This can then be followed through to establish that the person has a fear of meeting new people.

To establish how fearful they are, you could ask them to state on a scale of 1 to 10, where 1 is low and 10 high, how anxious they feel. If they answer with a 7, ask them where they would need to be on the scale to make it possible for them to join the class or group. They might then say 3. Now ask: *'What would you be doing to keep your anxiety at a 7?'* This might be followed by: *'Could you do more of that?'* Or: *'What would help you to reduce the anxiety level to a 5 or 6?'* If they have difficulty, you can help them by making some suggestions from which they can choose. Word the suggestions so that the person remains in control and does not feel that they are being imposed on them. For example: *'Another person who has similar difficulties tried ... and found it worked. What do you think?'* This allows the person to see that they are not the only one with this problem, that the suggestion has been successful with someone else and that you have given them the freedom to remain in control.

When an action has been discussed and agreed, say: *'Close your eyes and imagine that this has been put into place. How do you now feel and where are you on the scale?'* Sometimes they will reduce the number down by more than one number. Then follow up by asking: *'What else would help reduce your anxiety level number?'* Continue in this way until the level of anxiety goal has been achieved and the person feels they can cope with the situation.

Working out an action plan in this way gives both you and the person an indication of how high the anxiety level is, how far it needs to be reduced and an action plan to achieve the goal. The person feels they are in control and is likely to be more motivated to succeed.

Comment

This process can be carried out in many instances to ensure that individuals' basic needs are met. It enables them to become open to thinking about further growth and development or making changes. You do, however, need to take care over how you phrase the questions, so that the person feels they remain in control. Once the person feels comfortable – that their basic need has been met – they may well be able to acknowledge and work on essential changes to maintain or improve well-being.

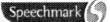

Strategy 3: Showing positive regard

Introduction

We all need to be treated with respect. Think about when a friend, another member of your family or a work colleague is disrespectful to you. They may not respect your interests, preferences, values, beliefs or opinions. How do you feel? You may become angry, want nothing to do with the person, feel downtrodden, become depressed, lose self-esteem, become fearful, dread going to work, and so on.

Mostly, people tend to respond accordingly, depending on how we treat them. If we treat them with a balance of respect and assertiveness then trust and a sense of positive regard will start to build.

How you could do this

Be genuine

Have the right thoughts in your mind when you approach or engage with the person you want to motivate. If your thoughts are genuine, so will your body language be, as will the message you convey.

If you are thinking: *'This is a waste of time. He'll just tell me to go away'* or *'I'm too busy to spend time persuading him to take part – awkward man!'*, this will show in your voice and your body language, and that is the message the person will receive. However, if you are thinking: *'It would be really helpful if John took part. He has a lot of experience and a lot to contribute to the group. He enjoys being useful and it will help him to make new friends'*, this too will show in your body language.

This is how Carl R. Rogers defines being genuine:

> In order to do this you need to ensure you have the right mindset before you engage with the person. Stop a moment, reflect and prepare to focus on the person and their needs – no matter how you may feel about dislikeable aspects of the person.
>
> (Rogers, 1967, p9)

This friendly, encouraging attitude needs to be maintained throughout your discussions. You need to show that:

- you see the person as your equal
- you are listening to and understanding what they say
- you respect their right to decide and act on any matters discussed
- they maintain control.

It can be very difficult to maintain positive regard for someone who is unpleasant or argumentative. The task is a balance between honesty and assertiveness, ensuring respect and fair treatment on both sides.

Ensure you provide the right environment and atmosphere

Different people and different aims require different approaches. Some people may feel comfortable with a formal approach, such as a handshake or a *'Good morning'*. Others may prefer a *'How's it going mate?'* or *'Hi, John! Got any plans for today?'*

You need to be adaptable and to judge whether the person is comfortable with a handshake, chatting over a cup of coffee, or prefers a formal setting, such as a private office, an interview room, a quiet corner in the lounge. They may like to chat while doing something, such as walking in the garden, shopping or a hobby.

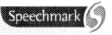

Why you are talking to the person will also need to be taken into account. Some personal matters will need a private setting, but not necessarily a formal environment such as an office. The person may be more comfortable and likely to respond in a private, casual setting. Let the person control the choice by asking: *'Where would you like us to chat – we could use the interview room, the coffee lounge or go out into the garden?'*

Give the person time to get their bearings, settle down and relax. You might:

- mention the surroundings

- talk about the weather

- make a complimentary remark (but be careful with this: it must be genuine – a false compliment used just for something to say can come across as patronising or being too familiar).

Showing affection

Without affection, life and motivation are diminished. Demonstrate this with a handshake and a word of congratulation: *'You've had your hair done. It really suits you'* or *'You are brave! I admire your spirit and determination.'*

Think of ways in which you show affection with your friends and relations. Make compliments, tell the person how well they are doing, celebrate small events with a cake or a card, or state your admiration for something they have achieved or overcome. Think about what might be appropriate in the environment in which you are working.

Do be aware of hugging or touching service users. If the situation makes a hug appropriate, ask for permission first. Not everyone likes to be touched.

Comment

In order to participate in activities and life generally, we need to feel that:

- we have some control over what happens to us

- our opinions, values, preferences, and so on are respected

- we can influence others and events.

In the absence of this, we feel that everything is being forced on us and we become passive or angry. These are very uncomfortable states to inhabit and often lead to depression and withdrawal or outbursts of aggression.

The first step in combating this is to show positive regard. This leads to helping the person see and make choices and feel that they can influence and have some control over their lives.

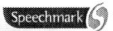

Strategy 4: Making a connection

Introduction

It is important to establish a rapport with the person you are supporting. This is essential for good communication. It enables dialogue and builds respect. To do this, you do not need to agree with the choices other people make. You may find their decisions or behaviour difficult to understand. This can give rise to feelings of irritation or anger about them.

Often, you may create rapport unconsciously. With some people you will find it easy to establish connections. With others you will need to work extremely hard to reach any understanding. You may have good 'people skills', but the person you are supporting may not. It is important to remember, as a carer or worker, that the responsibility for developing rapport lies with you. However, the prerogative to make choices remains with the person being cared for or supported. To make connections, we need to adopt useful behaviours.

How you could do this

Often, the responses we receive are not the ones we expect. The other person may interpret our approach in a way that we do not intend. It helps to be constantly aware of how communication works. How a person reacts gives us indications of how they are construing our behaviour. People respond in two ways:

- **Internally**, with thoughts and emotions. This includes previous experiences (both bad and good), cultural influences, feelings, expectations, pictures and sounds.

- **Externally**, which encompasses posture, gestures, expressions, tone of voice, touch, eye contact and sometimes skin tone.

An interaction may go something like as follows.

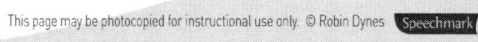

Peter approaches, smiling, and reaches out to shake hands. I respond internally, thinking: 'That is a false smile. He is only friendly when he wants something.' I turn away, ignoring the hand, and say 'Hello' to Morag.

Peter may have just wanted to be friendly. I have interpreted his intentions in the light of past experiences and what I thought was a false smile, and reacted accordingly.

Bearing this in mind, and the reaction that our own body language and behaviour can create in someone else's thoughts and behaviour, there are a number of techniques we can use to create rapport. You can try:

Matching body language. Often we do this automatically – smiling when the person smiles, looking serious when they do, and so on. We can also match their body posture, pitch and tone of voice, movements and breathing rhythms.

Matching language. This is using the same type of words and vocabulary as the other person uses in order to represent the world as they see it. Also, listen for and be aware whether they use words related to a particular sense, such as hearing, seeing or feeling, and reflect these back. You can pick these up from their statements: *'I feel ...', 'I can see ...', 'I sound as if ...'* Your answers might start: *'That **sounds** as if you ...', 'How does that make you **feel** ...?'* or *'What do you **see** happening ...?'*

Matching outcomes. Does what you are trying to do with the person match what they want? Do you both have the same goal? You might both want the person to feel better or resolve a difficulty. Have you both agreed on a desired outcome? If you try to manipulate them or force them to agree with you, they will probably continue to 'do their own thing' anyway, or adopt a resistant stance.

Matching learning style. The person may have a strong visual, hearing or 'doing' learning style. If you are giving information or explaining

 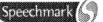

something, adopt what is appropriate. For a strong visual style, you might write down the information, do a simple sketch or demonstrate something. For a hearing style, perhaps read the information aloud or discuss it in detail with the person. For a 'doing' style, you might demonstrate and then encourage the person to have a go at doing whatever it is you have demonstrated.

Matching pace. The person might be reflective by nature and like time to think things through. Avoid rushing things – first establish some rapport and then gradually begin leading the person to a different state of mind. Let the person set the pace.

Showing a genuine interest in the person and their welfare. They will quickly become aware if your thoughts are elsewhere, you are filling in time or just going through a process. (Most settings entail going through established processes.) This will be reflected in their thoughts about you and in their body language and stop any ongoing dialogue or disclosures. We are all human and at times our minds can be deflected into something that is happening in our own lives and the rapport can be reduced or lost. When this happens, you need to focus your attention back quickly on to building connections. It is equally important that you reduce the intensity of rapport as you come to the end of your chat or session with the person. This helps to bring the engagement to an end, and avoids an abrupt ending.

Comment

You will probably use a mixture of the above when trying to engage with someone. It is important to remember that if one method does not work, you need to try another. Be careful when matching body language and vocabulary that doing so does not come across as mimicking the other person or they might think you are making fun of them. Don't overdo it! Neither would you want to match the posture of someone who is angry. That would only serve to escalate their anger. Instead, you could match their anger with the intensity of your listening and by using a non-threatening posture. You can then lead the person into a more relaxed state in which their difficulty can be explored.

 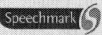

Strategy 5: Establishing values and beliefs

Introduction

Our values and beliefs drive our behaviour and give meaning to life. They define who we are and the personal rules we choose to live by. They motivate us. When they are aligned with what we are doing, we engage in life with enthusiasm. When not aligned, we lose our motivation and become unhappy.

The people with whom we live and associate normally share similar values. We feel comfortable and safe with them. Imagine being lifted out of an environment in which you feel safe and share values and being taken to a residential home or day centre or being placed with another family who are strangers. You have no choice about the staff or the other residents. This happens during a traumatic period in your life. You may have lost your parents, partner, home, a way of life, your health or the ability to look after yourself. How would you feel, think and behave? What fears would you have? What would be your reaction to staff, other residents or relatives who tried to get you to do things that were not aligned with your values and beliefs?

It is essential to establish what is important to the person you are trying to help to become motivated. This applies equally to an employee, a student or a friend.

Some people may not have consciously thought about their values and beliefs and may have difficulty verbalising them. They may say they are unhappy or have no motivation, but not know why. You will need to use prompts to help them think about and verbalise those beliefs and values.

How you could do this

To start the person thinking, provide suggestions or a list of values from which they can choose. Your list might include the following.

 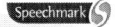

Friendships	Honesty	Having fun
Being independent	Spirituality	Privacy
Maintaining dignity	Respect	Kindness
Achievement	Risk	Security
Creativity	Knowledge	Leadership
Fairness	Choice	Growth
Compassion	Integrity	Loyalty
Discipline	Dedication	Flexibility

Encourage the person to list (or state) up to 10 things they value and write alongside each one why that quality is important to them. Examples might be:

Independence: because it allows me to do the things I want to do.

Knowledge: because I believe knowledge is the key to success and happiness.

You can help individuals identify their values by asking them to recall a time when things were going well for them. Then ask:

'What were you doing?'

'What inspired you at the time?'

'What value or quality were you being true to?'

'Do you still feel the same now?'

Next, ask them to think of a time when things were not going well for them and then ask:

'What were you doing?'

'How did you feel at the time?'

'What value were you not being true to?'

You could also ask:

'What values would you best like to be known or remembered for?'

Comment

The outcome can be recorded in personal records, in a personal diary or on a 'My Values' sheet to be kept in a folder as a reminder. The process can easily be adapted for working with groups.

Some individuals may have beliefs and values which no longer support them in their daily lives. You may need to spend time helping them evaluate their current usefulness.

 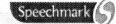

Strategy 6: Raising awareness

Introduction

The person may or may not be aware of what is causing their predicament or that they have a problem. They could be in denial and unwilling to face it. Perhaps they are difficult to engage or they may be withdrawn and uncommunicative. An approach may be to raise awareness of the situation and the possibility of change. The aim at this stage is to raise doubt and increase the person's perception of the risks and problems that flow from their current behaviour.

Avoid using scare tactics. This may activate or increase denial as a way of dealing with something they lack confidence about or do not know how to deal with. Also, refrain from trying to provide or explore answers. The person must first acknowledge the problem and the possibility of change.

How you could do this

Talk to the person and ask questions which help explore the situation. These should be dropped into the conversation in a matter-of-fact manner. Use open questions that cannot be answered with 'Yes' or 'No'. These will usually begin with 'What?', 'How?', 'When?' or 'Where?' Avoid the conversation becoming an interrogation by using different approaches. For example:

'Tell me more about ... What do you think will be the outcome?'

'Can you describe ...? How will you be affected?'

'I'd like to know more about ... '

'Will that create more difficulties for you? Where will you go?'

'That's interesting. When should you stop doing this?'

Occasionally summarise or ask a closed question that provides a 'Yes' or 'No' answer to clarify and reinforce points. For example:

'When you are feeling threatened, you lock yourself in your room. Is that correct?'

'Do you think that if you continue living in this way you will become more depressed?'

'When you feel angry you release your anger by picking an argument with someone. Have I got that right?'

Enable the person to relate their story. Keep the conversation slow and relaxed and use body language to show interest by nodding, maintaining good eye contact, leaning forwards and saying things like: *'Go on'*, *'What did you do?'* and *'That's interesting'*. Allow silent periods and avoid trying to interpret or being judgemental. At this stage you are trying to raise awareness, bring the problem to the surface and enable the person to acknowledge it and accept that there might be an opportunity to make changes.

Comment

Conversations can be followed up with providing information leaflets and/or further discussion to explore issues around the problem. These might include symptoms of depression, addiction or whatever the concern is, and about how continuing to ignore the matter might affect the person in the future. Often just explaining information and talking about concerns can raise interest in the possibility that change can happen. However, do be careful not to overdo the discussion or overload the person with too much information in one go. They may not yet be motivated to make changes, but some interest has been aroused. And you may need to return to this stage in the process a number of times, using awareness-raising tactics, before the person is able to move on to the next stage.

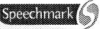

Strategy 7: Using active listening skills

Introduction

Listening to the person, observation and reflection skills are essential to help create rapport and start the process of building and increasing the motivation to change. We may jump in and quickly try to fix the problem or we may make assumptions about the person and listen only to things which support these suppositions. It is our natural instinct to interrupt by asking questions and to start offering advice, producing an action plan, arguing and contradicting, and trying to persuade the person to take the advice we offer – all of this without hearing what is tentatively being said, reflecting on our understanding or exploring the whole situation. We may even get annoyed because they do not do what we see as a solution. The result is that our assessment is inaccurate, the person backs off, feeling we do not understand, and becomes even more resistant and intransigent. The first priority is to listen, observe and check meaning, avoiding any impulse to give advice or provide solutions.

How you could do this

Often, when a person approaches us, we have our own or the workplace goals in mind. Our thoughts may be focused on another activity and the pressure of completing other tasks. It may be necessary to make an appointment with the person for a time when, and in a place where, you can listen to and give them your full attention without interruptions.

Active listening involves taking an interest in what the person has to say and respecting their self-knowledge and viewpoint. We may see things which the person cannot, or which they may not yet be aware of, but they remain the expert on their own wants, desires, choices, beliefs, behaviours and development. To find out about these things we need to listen, draw them out and understand their viewpoint. To ensure that we do understand and have not got it wrong, we need to check our interpretation of what has been said. You can do this in four ways: by asking open-ended questions, by making statements and affirmations and by summarising.

1 Open-ended questions

These are questions which cannot be answered with *'Yes'* or *'No'*. If I ask: *'Do you feel depressed?'*, I will get a *'Yes'* or *'No'* answer. What 'depressed' means to the person and what I understand it to mean may be quite different. If I ask: *'Can you describe how you feel?'*, I am more likely to get a detailed answer that gives me a more accurate understanding of what the person is experiencing. Also, open-ended questions enable the person to feel in control of whatever is bothering them. It is happening to them and they are the expert on the subject. Closed questions tend to set up you, the support worker, as being the expert and can lead to the person expecting you to provide the answers or to them becoming more resistant to any changes that might be needed.

The manner in which questions are asked determines the type of answers you receive. As previously stated, most begin with *'How'*, *'What'* or *'When'*. It is usually best to minimise the use of *'Why'* as this can lead the person into starting to analyse their situation rather than stating it. Other typical open questions are:

> *'In what way is that a problem for you?'*
>
> *'What do you want to achieve?'*
>
> *'How would you like things to be different?'*
>
> *'When will you do that?'*
>
> *'Tell me how did you cope when you had all this to do?'*
>
> *'How did you manage to do that?'*
>
> *'What traits helped you to achieve that?'*
>
> *'How did you maintain hope during this period?'*

2 Making statements

> *'So, you are unsure if the group would benefit you.'*
>
> *'You're wondering if ...'*
>
> *'Before taking part, you want to know ...'*

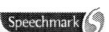

Making a statement, rather than asking a question gives the person the opportunity to expand on or clarify the meaning of what they have said. Asking questions such as: *'Do you want to know if the group would benefit you?'* or *'Do you want me to ...?'* can tend to interrupt, stop the flow and receive a *'Yes'* or *'No'* reply. When we make a statement, the inflexion, tone of voice and emphasis we use is different, making it more likely the person will expand on what they have said so far.

3 Affirmations

Making an affirmation needs to be done with sincerity in a way that supports and promotes the person's feelings of being in control. Do this by providing compliments, statements of appreciation and understanding. Acknowledge the difficulties the person has experienced and validate their feelings. Emphasise experiences that demonstrate strength and success. For example:

'That must have been very difficult for you. It shows terrific strength of character.'

'That's a really good idea.'

'That was a really big step. I would have thought twice about doing all that in one go.'

'You show remarkable resourcefulness to have coped so well with all the stress you have been experiencing.'

'You are setting a really good example of how to cope under extreme pressure. Your family must be very proud of you.'

Always focus on strengths and attributes. Reframe negative statements into affirmations:

'Despite how you were feeling, you did the exercises on three days this week. How did you manage to do that?'

'Although you have reservations, you are willing to try an experiment. That shows determination.'

4 Summarising

Summarising confirms what has been said, shows that you have been listening and prepares the person to move on. Use summaries at intervals to recap, or at the beginning and end of sessions. A major benefit of summarising is that it helps people to feel understood. Other uses include drawing the person's attention to something or highlighting the pros and cons of what has been covered so far. It also helps with keeping track of the conversation. Often, summaries will lead to more disclosures. Here is an example:

'So far, my understanding is that the benefits you derive from attending the taster course include: a gain in confidence, most days you feel good, you have a sense of purpose, you enjoy the learning and the company of the other students. And you think you would like to do a qualification course. On the other hand, you have some bad days when you feel depressed and it is all too much; you think it is all pointless and that the other students and the tutor think you are stupid and you have no chance of gaining a qualification.'

If the summary serves to move the discussion forwards, this indicates progress. If it results in repetition, the person may feel they have not been correctly understood or have mixed thoughts or contradictory ideas (see 'Discrepancies' overleaf) about something and feel ambivalent.

During the process of using this approach, avoid offering solutions or advice. Instead, focus on what the person is saying and mirror some of their body language.

Observation

Around 90 per cent of communication is non-verbal; that is, through body language. To understand the other person's viewpoint, you need to notice and reflect understanding of non-verbal reactions – often, people will say one thing, but their body language indicates another meaning. This will include your understanding of:

 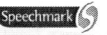

- facial expressions – frowns, raised eyebrows, smiles, grimaces, etc

- tone and volume of voice

- pauses, silences, blushing, paleness

- ambiguous or generalised statements that need clarification

- body movements, posture and rhythms

- indications of feelings.

You need to make clear your understanding of these reactions in a way that enables the person to expand on or clarify the meaning. For example:

'You say you will rejoin the group, but am I right in thinking you are not entirely happy with ...?'

'I sense that there is something else you would like to talk about.'

'You are brave to do this, but I'm wondering if you ...'

Discrepancies

Often, people make statements or do things which are inconsistent with their beliefs or what they say are their long-term goals. They then feel uncomfortable about, or are unhappy carrying out, the agreed actions, or they lack the motivation to do so. Pointing out and making them aware of these discrepancies is helpful in enabling them to understand why they are stuck. It helps them to begin to be motivated to do something about it. Some examples might be:

'You say you feel lonely and yet you stay in your room rather than come down to the lounge. What do you think will be the outcome if you continue to do this?'

'How do you see your continued use of alcohol in this way affecting your ability to complete this course?'

The aim is to draw out the inconsistencies and enable the person to recognise and acknowledge the consequence of their current behaviour. You can then gently help them to explore their concerns. This, in turn, can lead to them expressing a desire for change and to realign their actions with their beliefs and goals.

Comment

Listening to people and observing them without jumping in and providing solutions is not easy. Neither is checking their understanding and phrasing statements and questions in a way that draws them out and puts them on a path that leads to them being motivated to make change. It is an acquired skill that needs a lot of practice. It is also a skill you need to use throughout all stages of the change process.

 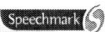

Strategy 8: Providing information

Introduction

Providing information can prompt hope and the motivation to make changes. Someone may be stuck in the idea that they cannot change, may have tried a number of things and may now have given up hope. This may be due to a lack of information or knowledge. For example:

- A person may become motivated when they learn about how others, who share similar problems, have succeeded.

- A service user may become motivated to exercise when informed about the benefits of doing so and the consequences of not doing so.

- A resident may become motivated to try joining a group to break her isolation when she knows the options available to her.

It is equally true that other people will become more resistant to change when given information. They may feel it is being forced on them or not want to know. Classic examples are some people who smoke, have other addictions, are excessively overweight, have behavioural problems, or act in a bullying way. There are many actions that are helpful or unhelpful and we need to express these facts. In these cases, to lessen the resistance, the way in which the information is given is very important.

In motivational interviewing, there is a process called 'prefacing' which can be used in these situations. The method entails expressing 'uncertainty' as to whether the information will be useful. This provides the person with total autonomy and leaves them feeling free to decide what is helpful for them. You can then ask whether they think anything you have said would help. The idea is that the 'uncertainty' of this tentative approach may spark some interest, which can be followed up by promoting thoughts of making changes.

How you could do this

There are various approaches to this. Here are a few ways in which you could start:

'This may or may not interest you. Some people in your situation ...'

'I don't know if this will apply to you, but ...'

'A thought occurred to me that might be of interest to you ...'

'Some people have told me that doing ... can make things worse. Have you tried it?'

'I'm not sure about this, but ...'

'Can you tell me if it would interest you to ...?'

'A friend in similar circumstances to you tried ...'

'Only someone in your position would know if this would help.'

'I would value your opinion on whether or not ...'

You then go on to explain what you have in mind. You end the approach by asking the person what they think of the idea:

'What do you think of that?'

'Do you think that's a good idea?'

'I wonder if that would appeal to you?'

'I'm not sure if it's worth trying?'

You may have to allow the person time to think about the idea. This might mean returning to the subject a few times to answer questions and give further information before moving on to the next stage, when the person begins expressing a desire to make the change.

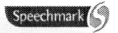

Comment

When information is given in this way with a tone of 'uncertainty', a resistant person is more likely to accept it. It helps to reinforce their feelings of control and freedom of action. When giving information, the tone should always be one of informing, not of persuading.

Strategy 9: Building self-esteem

Introduction

For some people, before they can think about making changes, the most important thing may be to build self-esteem. When we have good self-esteem, we can make choices about how we run our lives and set goals, believing that we can achieve them. If we have low self-esteem, we do not feel in control of our life, confidence ebbs away, and we lose belief in our ability to achieve. The result is that motivation is destroyed. Therefore, the first task may be to build the individual's self-esteem.

How you could do this

Give compliments and state your appreciation. This can be very helpful in breaking down barriers and making connections.

This does not always mean that you increase the number of compliments you give. Too many can come across as patronising and false. The gesture must be genuine – otherwise it will be counterproductive. Quality, not quantity, is the guide.

Someone with low self-esteem is more likely to benefit from praise made in private – it comes across as more personal. Also, avoid 'going over the top', or giving it in a rushed – 'by-the-way' – manner or when the person is in a very negative state of mind: these are times when the person is more likely to reject praise and not benefit from it.

It is better to understate compliments slightly until the person has built up their self-esteem and they feel more comfortable accepting them. They are also more likely to accept the compliments.

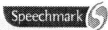

Make eye contact

The person may lower their eyes or try to avoid eye contact by looking away. When you make eye contact, it shows your interest and respect for the person. Also, state the person's name and repeat it occasionally. This reaffirms that they are not ignored and are acknowledged and respected as a person. Think about times when you have been ignored or your name has been left out of something repeatedly. How did you feel? This feeling will be magnified by someone with low self-esteem. Keep it simple: *'Good morning, Dorothy!'* or *'Would you like to join us, Dorothy?'*, and so on. Be careful not to overdo it, though.

Be specific

'You made a good job of the display, Bob' is a general comment. It is more effective to state specifically why you think it was a good job. *'You made a great flower display in the entrance, Bob. Many of the visitors remarked on the beautiful colours. It really helped to create a friendly and welcoming atmosphere. Thank you!'*

Use 'I' statements

Saying *'I enjoyed our chat'* rather than *'That was a nice chat'*, or *'I appreciate your help laying the tables'* rather than *'You were a big help today'* personalises the statement and shows your personal appreciation. It is also helpful in building a relationship with the person.

Help the person identify their good points

Do this by helping the person explore and make reinforcing statements about:

- their achievements in life – both past and present
- challenges they have faced in the past and have overcome
- talents they have – however small
- skills they have
- what you and other people value and appreciate about them.

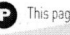

Some examples might be:

'Your sense of humour cheers me up.'

'You keep the group focused and on target. That is a real help to me. Thank you!'

'You looked after your mother when she was ill. That must have been difficult while holding down a job and looking after two children. It shows you have determination, good organisational skills and a caring nature.'

Activity diaries

Encourage and assist the person to record a daily diary of what they have done, what gave them pleasure and satisfaction and what they achieved. Remind the person that a small task completed, a minor problem solved or something done that they have been putting off are all successes. This helps to change the emphasis from focusing on everything that has not been done to acknowledging what has been accomplished.

Encourage the use of 'me' time

This is time spent for personal enjoyment. It is time the person sets aside to do something that benefits them and may or may not include other people. Agreeing to have 'me' time is an acknowledgement to ourselves that we are worth it. The reasons people give for not planning and using 'me' time may include statements such as:

'I'm not worth it.'

'I've no idea what I would do.'

'I couldn't do that. It's too selfish and self-indulgent.'

'I'd feel guilty.'

'I don't have time for that.'

'I'd feel silly.'

 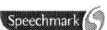

You will need to help individuals challenge these thoughts and support them as they carry out their plans or explore what they could do during their 'me' time.

'Me' time may include such pursuits as:

Sitting in the garden	Having coffee with a friend
Going for a walk	Drawing or painting
Reading a novel	Having a facial
Gardening	Going to a class
Swimming	Playing basketball
Listening to music	Doing yoga
Going to see a show	Dancing
Writing a diary	Watching a favourite television show

Challenge negative attitudes

The person may have formed a habit of regularly making negative statements about themselves such as:

'I'm no good at ...'

'I can't do ...'

'I always fail ...'

'I'm hopeless at ...'

'Nobody likes me.'

'I don't have any skills.'

Gently but firmly help the person challenge these statements by pointing out positives, such as:

'That's not true! Yesterday you cooked some delicious cakes.'

'Why do you think that? Earlier you helped Peter write a letter to his son. He was very grateful for your help.'

'You have demonstrated a number of skills today. You organised the rota, sorted out the library books to be returned and did a really super poster for the quiz tomorrow night. That has been a real help to me. You have lots of skills.'

Comment

Indications of poor self-esteem show in many ways, providing us with clues about how the person might be feeling. Take note of their body language. Look for clues in what the person says, how they say it and how they dress.

- Are they wearing bright or subdued colours?

- Are there a lot of negative comments, self-criticism and apologies?

- How do they get on with you and other people? Are they exceptionally shy and quiet, or pushy? What does this say about them?

- Observe their posture. Do they tend to adopt a hunched, inward posture and avoid eye contact?

- Do they appear sad, anxious or angry or reveal signs of feeling shame, guilt or inadequacy?

- Do they have difficulty speaking out and avoid opportunities or do they show signs of tension or fatigue?

 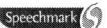

Strategy 10: Responding to resistance

Introduction

If a person displays resistant behaviour, it is a sure sign that you need to change your approach. You probably need to listen more and reflect your understanding of what you hear (see Strategy 7: 'Using active listening skills'). If they respond by giving more information, or making statements that indicate thoughts about the possibility of change, then progress is being made.

Thomas Gordon (1970, pp41–7, 108–17, 321–7) listed the actions which may interfere with this forwards movement. He called them 'roadblocks'. They include:

Ordering	Advising	Moralising
Directing	Providing solutions	Preaching
Commanding	Making suggestions	Telling service users their duty
Warning	Arguing	Judging
Threatening	Lecturing	Criticising
Agreeing	Persuading with logic	Disagreeing
Approving	Shaming	Blaming
Praising	Ridiculing	Name calling
Interpreting	Questioning	Withdrawing
Analysing	Probing	Distracting
Humouring	Changing the subject	

Indulging in any of these actions is likely to encourage resistance and result in a dead end: particularly when you are trying to arouse interest in the need for change or the person has just begun to consider making a change. For example:

Service user:	*'I didn't touch her handbag.'*
Worker:	*'You were there at the time and you have stolen stuff before.'* (blaming and judging)
Service user:	*'Why blame me? There were other people there too! Caroline regularly takes stuff that doesn't belong to her.'*
Worker:	*'I'm going to keep a close eye on you. Lying doesn't help. Don't go in the lounge in future. Your behaviour is disgraceful and you are heading for disaster.'* (threatening, accusing, ordering, blaming, lecturing)

Be aware of the effect of your own behaviour. If you find yourself becoming caught up in an argument, or someone becomes defensive, change your behaviour in order to elicit a different response.

How you could do this

Avoiding arguing

It is very easy to find yourself arguing against something you strongly disagree with and feel you need to correct. You might state a different viewpoint and then the service user challenges the accuracy of what you say, questions your expertise or becomes hostile. A way to avoid this is to use 'Socratic-type questions'. Socrates was an educator in Greece in the fifth century BC, who taught by asking questions which led his pupils to work out the answers for themselves. This technique needs to be combined with listening and reflection skills. The purpose is to challenge the accuracy of the person's thinking, raise their awareness and guide

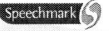

them to presenting the arguments for change themselves. Here are some suggestions:

- To get them to think more about what they are saying, or to prove it, use 'tell me more' questions to clarify their viewpoint:

  'What does that mean?'

  'Can you give me any examples?'

  'In what way does that relate to what you want to do?'

  'Can you tell me how that would help you?

- To probe the basis and assumptions on which they are basing their statement:

  'What would happen if ...?'

  'Can you prove or disprove that assumption?'

  'Do you agree or disagree with ...?'

  'Can you explain ...?'

- To check their reasoning:

  'What makes you think that?'

  'What's the evidence to support that?'

  'What do you think causes ...?'

  'Why do you think that happens?'

- To show there are other, equally valid viewpoints:

  'What would be an alternative way of looking at this?'

  'What are the strengths and weaknesses of ...?'

  'How would your partner see this?'

  'Someone else might approach this by ... What do you think of that?'

- To explore consequences:

  'What would happen if …?'

  'How would that affect …?'

  'How does that fit with …?'

  'How could … be used to …?'

Asking too many questions can come across as aggressive. When there is high resistance, keep the questions to a minimum and rely on the use of listening and reflection skills.

Responding to interruptions

Sometimes the person may interrupt or talk over you before waiting for an appropriate pause. They may be trying to dominate the conversation, divert it away from the issue or they may be showing interest. You can view this either as the person being disruptive or difficult or as an opportunity to gain more information about their viewpoint.

If you believe it is a diversion, try changing the focus by either briefly summarising your understanding so far or asking one or two Socratic-type questions. The interruption might also indicate discrepancies between the person's present concerns and the purpose of the interview or their longer-term goals.

Dealing with denial

The person does not acknowledge the problem, cooperate, accept responsibility or take advice. They may blame someone else, disagree with or refute suggestions, make excuses, or minimise the issue by suggesting that it is all being exaggerated and that they are not affected by it, and that you are being pessimistic. There may be a lack of desire or willingness to change or they state that they have no intention of changing.

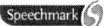

You are likely to increase resistance by using any of the 'roadblock' methods listed above. Start by trying to get an understanding of the person's reasons for staying the same. Use appropriate Socratic-type questions and reflective listening skills (see Strategy 18: 'Using reflective listening skills to roll with resistance') to do this. Reinforce their feelings of personal control and raise their awareness of any inconsistencies in their thinking, values and behaviour. The aim is to make them feel safe, so that they can begin to explore the notion of making changes.

Responding to being ignored

The person appears not to be listening, does not respond to questions, gives a response that ignores what has been asked, sidetracks or changes the direction of the conversation. This can easily result in you feeling angry, becoming impatient, giving up or not bothering with the person. Service users can become highly skilled at sidetracking or ignoring suggestions for help.

One approach may be to offer your perception as a concern. A typical lead-in might be:

> 'Jane, we have talked about ... There's one more thing that I would like to discuss, if you don't mind? I have noticed that ... I'm concerned that you might be trying to do too much and it's affecting your health. What do you think?'

Always end the observation or concern by asking for the service user's view of what you have said. Any comment they make can then be followed by more listening and reflecting and some further questions.

Bear in mind that some people may be able to focus and concentrate only for short periods of time and have a very limited attention span. They may not be deliberately ignoring you, but have just forgotten or lost track of the conversation.

Disagreeing with a decision

There may be times when you disagree with a decision someone has made. You can state this as a discrepancy and/or concern:

> 'Tim, you have stated your intention to go to the party with Tom and Peter. Previously you said that it's when you go out together that you drink excessively. Peter regularly spikes your drink because he thinks it's funny. It's when you drink that you become argumentative and aggressive and, in the past, have hit Susan when you returned home. I'm concerned it will happen again. Susan has made it clear she will leave if it does. How does this fit with you saying you love Susan and want to marry her?'

Occasionally, a person may feel deeply ashamed or pained and unable to talk about something. They may want to, but just cannot vocalise it. You can ask them if they would like to write it down or draw it. They could also try talking or writing about themselves in the third person – that is, substituting 'she/he' for 'I'. If none of these approaches works, try offering the person some set times to meet. Make it clear that during these periods they can remain silent or talk, if they wish, about their problem. You are just being there for them. Keep the periods short as it is very difficult to remain with someone in this way without talking to them, to help them bear their shame, guilt or pain.

One person I used this tactic with had to sit with her back to me at first. Then, after a few sessions, she was able to face me. Next, she was able to do some drawings about how she was feeling. She was then able to depict what was causing her to feel this way. This led to her beginning to vocalise what was happening that was troubling her.

Comment

Be careful, when asking Socratic-type questions, that you do not allow a tone of sarcasm, criticism or challenge to creep into your voice. The questions need to be posed in an enquiring way that indicates you are trying to understand the person's viewpoint.

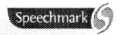

Miller and Rollnick state in their book *Motivational Interviewing* that:

> In expressing resistance, the client is probably rehearsing a script
> that has been played out many times before. There is an expected
> role for you to play – one that has been acted by others in the past.
> Your lines are predictable. If you speak these same lines, as others
> have done, the script will come to the same conclusion as before.

(Miller & Rollnick,1991, p111)

Those predictable scripts normally involve the use of Thomas Gordon's
'roadblocks'. You can change that script by taking a different approach.

SECTION 2

Encouraging individuals to consider change (Contemplation)

The person may have some awareness of the problem, but is still not motivated to do anything about it. They may think about it and decide against doing anything. Decisions are put off and action is avoided. There is a good deal of procrastination, talking about the problem, expressing concern, looking for reassurance and wanting to find out more. They want to change, but are still resistant to doing so. They may feel anxious about losing the security of their current familiar lifestyle, and fear either what the changes will bring or failing again. They may be looking for absolute certainty or for the problem to disappear while they are thinking about it. It is easy to become stuck in this position and be forever contemplating, but never taking, action.

The role of the worker here is to help tip the balance towards change and commitment to it. This means focusing on strategies to reinforce the reasons for change, the risks of not changing and the person's belief in being able to implement change.

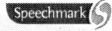

Strategy 11: Using a motivational balance sheet

Introduction

The *Concise Oxford Dictionary* (Pearson, 2011) gives the meaning of 'ambivalent' as 'having mixed feelings or opinions about something or someone'. Life often places us in situations that present us with difficult choices. We feel pulled in opposing directions by different emotions. The issues run round and round in a circle inside our head in a never-ending debate. This leaves us stuck in a state of indecision and inaction (ambivalence) which can go on for months or years. A sure sign that we are caught in a state of being ambivalent is when we keep putting off to another day taking action about an important matter. We may be aware there is a problem, but we lack the motivation to do anything about it. Before a service user is able to move forwards to planning any action, these feelings of 'ambivalence' need to be addressed.

How you could do this

For the person to become 'unstuck', you need to help them explore both the forces 'driving' and those 'restraining' change. If the balance is even, the person will remain stuck (see Figure 2).

Each of the forces will have a different weight value. Both 'driving' and 'restraining' elements need to be fully explored, otherwise the forces against change are likely to emerge again later and hinder progress. Individuals need to know how to deal with any losses that will occur. Also, during exploration some of the 'restraining' elements may be able to be converted to 'driving' elements, thus tipping the balance (see Figure 3).

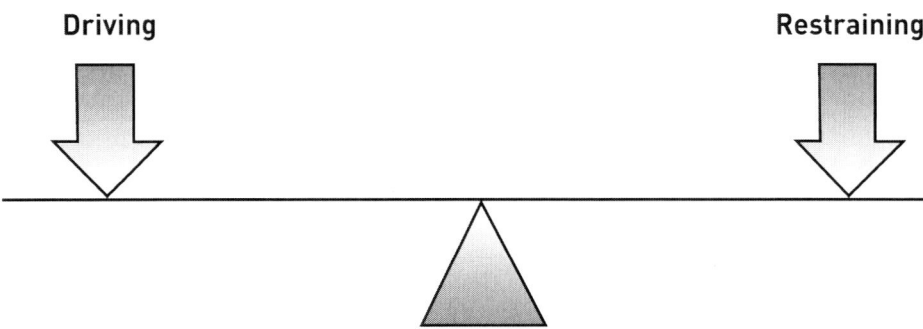

Figure 2 Evenly balanced 'driving' and 'restraining' forces

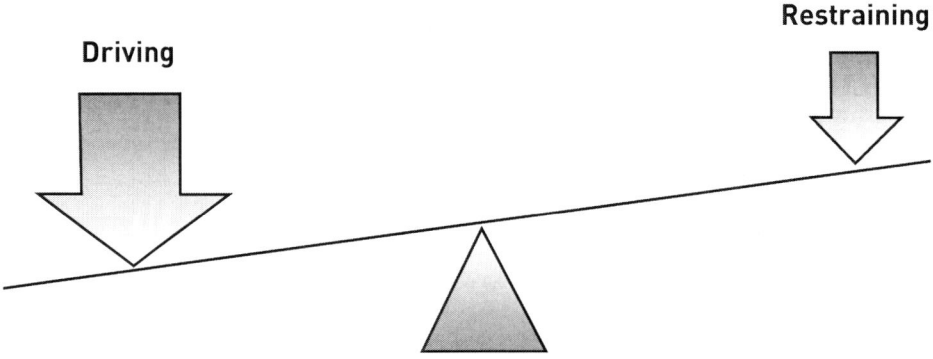

Figure 3 Balance weighed towards 'driving' change

People do not change just because of logic. Logically, change may make sense, but it is not what drives people to change. Logically, we may acknowledge that it makes sense to do something, but we do not do it until we are emotionally compelled to do so. This makes it essential to look not just at the logical reasons for making changes, but also at the underlying emotional motivation to drive these changes.

We must also be careful not to put our own weighing up of or influence on the importance of any factors. To do this we need to use open questions and reflective listening skills to bring out what is important to the person both currently and in the future. By using these skills and summarising, we can help the person become aware of any discrepancies between their current behaviour and what they want in the future.

While exploring the 'driving' and 'restraining' forces, it is essential that the focus is on exploring and understanding the person's world. The process can be carried out in four stages as described below.

Stage 1

Establish with the person what behaviour they are unhappy with or feel ambivalent about. Once this is clear, enquire how they would like this to be different in six months or a year from now, as appropriate. A typical lead-in might be:

'Describe to me how you would like things to be in six months' time.'

Follow up this by using open questions to explore their vision. Ensure that your enquiries are from a positively desired perspective. An example might be:

'Imagine that in six months' time this has actually happened. Take your time, close your eyes if you like, and conjure it up in your imagination. Now tell me: what are you thinking about yourself?

What are other people saying to you?

Describe how you feel.

How much do you want to achieve this goal?'

Stage 2

Now ask the person how much they want to make the changes necessary to attain this goal and how confident they feel in their ability to achieve it. Mark this on simple 1–10 rating scale charts like the ones shown in Figures 4 and 5.

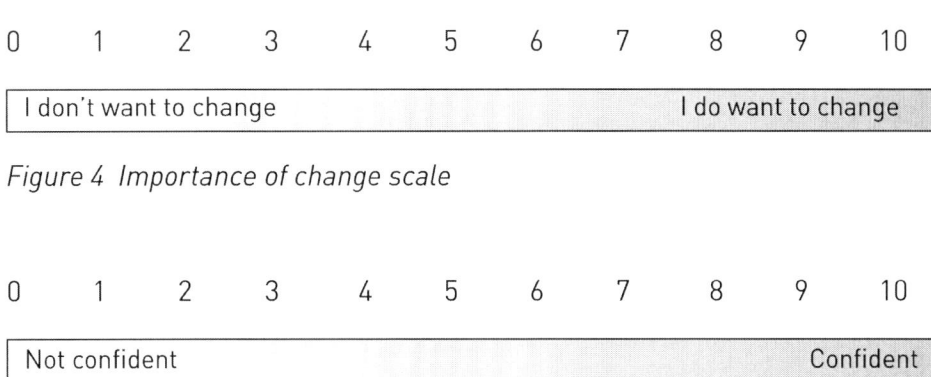

| 0 | 1 | 2 | 3 | 4 | 5 | 6 | 7 | 8 | 9 | 10 |

| I don't want to change | I do want to change |

Figure 4 Importance of change scale

| 0 | 1 | 2 | 3 | 4 | 5 | 6 | 7 | 8 | 9 | 10 |

| Not confident | Confident |

Figure 5 Confidence in ability scale

Stage 3

Using a balance sheet like that shown in Figure 6, invite the person to write down the reasons why they want to change (driving forces) and the reasons why they want to stay as they are (restraining forces).

Strength of reason (1–10)	Restraining forces (Reasons to stay the same)	Driving forces (Reasons to make changes)	Strength of reason (1–10)
Total:			**Total:**

Figure 6   Balance sheet

The column 'Driving forces' will contain what the person wants for the future and things related to what they dislike about their current situation. The 'Restraining forces' column will contain what they like about their current situation. Ensure that the columns include factors that are both internal (fears, emotions, benefits, doubts, concerns, etc) and external (practical obstacles). Ask the person to give each entry a strength-of-reason number between 1 and 10, where 1 is a weak reason and 10 is a strong reason.

A completed sheet might look like Figure 7.

Strength of reason (1–10)	Restraining forces (Reasons to stay the same)	Driving forces (Reasons to make changes)	Strength of reason (1–10)
9	Going out drinking helps me relax	Be able to focus and concentrate and not upset others on the course with my behaviour	5
8	Meet people		
6	Helps me forget my worries	Will be able to complete the course	7
9	Have fun	My parents will be proud of me	5
9	If I don't go drinking with my friends, they won't want to know me. I'll lose them	Will be able to keep my job	8
		Will be able to pay off my debts	5
		My girlfriend will stay with me	9
Total: 41			**Total: 39**

Figure 7 Example of a completed balance sheet

Then draw out the reasons by asking questions such as:

'Why do you think what you are doing now is a problem? In what ways does it concern you?'

'What do you think concerns your tutor/girlfriend/parents/boss/other people on the course?'

'How do you feel about what you are doing?'

'What concerns you about changing this?'

'How do you see changing your behaviour helping you get what you really want?'

'Tell me, how would this help you achieve what you want?'

'What reasons do you see for making changes?'

'How would changing make life better for you?'

Stage 4

You can now help the person review their balance sheet and explore whether any of the driving forces can be increased in strength or additional ones added and any restraining force reduced. For example, friends are obviously important to the person in Figure 7. He could be asked: *'You have said that having friends is important to you. Tell me, what effect do you think your changed behaviour will have on the other people on the course?'* The answer might be: *'I would get on better with them and make new friends.'* This could then be added as an additional driving force for change, with a rating. Also, he might consider reducing the rating given to his fear of losing his drinking friends.

Other restraining forces that might be reduced or eliminated could be *'Going out drinking helps me relax'* and *'Helps me forget my worries'* or *'Have fun'*. For example: *'You say going out drinking helps you relax. What else have you done in the past that has helped you relax?'* The reply might

be: '*I used to go swimming with the guys from work. We often had competitions. I liked that. It was good fun.*' This might then be followed up as an alternative to going drinking, reducing the strength of the 'Going out drinking' and 'Have fun' restraining forces and adding to the driving forces for change.

Alternatively, you could raise the person's awareness of the discrepancy between constantly going out drinking and the influence this has on his behaviour and his vision of the future. For example: '*Tell me, how do you see going out drinking every night fits with you wanting to complete your qualification, keep your job and maintain your relationship with your girlfriend?*' If one direction does not lead anywhere, you can always change course.

Sometimes the person will start to make statements such as '*I see that I must ...*', '*It's becoming clear that ...*' or '*I can't go on the way I have been doing ...*', or give other signs that they are starting to see a way forward. These signal the start of the motivation to change. To help the person build on and develop these indications, also see Strategy 12: 'Building motivation to change'.

Comment

The idea is to destabilise the status quo and enable the person to start seeing a way forward. They may also now re-evaluate the importance and confidence scales (Figures 4 and 5). Once the 'driving' forces have been increased, they are highly likely to move upwards, showing increased motivation and confidence.

Strategy 12: Building motivation to change

Introduction

When the person begins to make statements that indicate dissatisfaction with their current situation, or that they are thinking of changing, it is necessary to draw out a shared definition of the problem. It is essential to do this before rushing on to explore solutions. If you move on too quickly, resistance to change will start to re-emerge.

How you could do this

In the language used by the person, there will be a mixture of statements: some that appear to sustain the status quo and others that indicate a desire for change. Listen for and reinforce those statements which focus on change. Acknowledge, but give only very limited attention to, talk which opposes change. This is a process which allows the person to persuade themself they need to change. To do this, use a combination of questioning, listening, reflecting and summarising. (See Strategy 7: 'Using active listening skills'.)

The person may begin to make comments or show aspects of body language which suggest concerns about what they are doing and the effect of this on others and themselves: *'I become aggressive when I drink a lot. I say something nasty and she gets upset. It's not fair'* or *'It worries me that my drinking every night is affecting my relationships at home and at work.'*

When such statements are made, reflect back the meaning of what has been said: *'So, you are worried about the effects your drinking has on relationships both at home and at work.'* As the person hears their own words repeated, this will increase their motivation to change, and they frequently follow those words with something like: *'I should do something about it.'* The aim is then to move this on towards the person stating that they do want to do something about it. Do this by asking something like:

'What would it mean to others if you did change your drinking habits?'

'How would you benefit if you did change?'

'On a scale of 1 to 10, how important is it for you to change?'

'What would need to happen to move your motivation up one on the scale?'

These questions also help to draw out the reason why the person wants to change. You might introduce a driving and restraining balance sheet at this stage (see Strategy 11: 'Using a motivational balance sheet'): these questions would then be used during this process. Finally, the person needs to state their intention to do something about changing and how confident they feel about being able to achieve their goal. Questions that help to draw this out include:

'What makes you think you will change?'

'Why is it important that you do change?'

'How confident do you feel about making the change?'

Comment

The desire to change often comes from the person becoming aware of the discrepancies between their current behaviour, their values and/or what they really want. Using listening skills to pick up on these, and carefully placed questions, reflections and summaries to highlight them, is essential for the person to become unstuck. As indicated above, do keep in mind that the person needs to acknowledge that there is a problem, agree what the problem is as they see it, and state their intention to change, before moving on to explore any solutions. The fact that there is a problem may be obvious to you and the person's relatives, friends or carers, but not necessarily to the person him- or herself. Also, the person may view the problem differently, which will require different solutions.

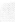 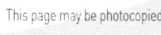

Strategy 13: Increasing belief in ability to change

Introduction

There are times when people feel that they want to make changes, but doubt whether they will be able to. Sometimes these doubts grow, dampening determination until people lose faith in their ability and give up on any hope of changing. However, if they become more confident in their ability, their desire and motivation to make the change becomes greater. They are more likely to take a first step towards achieving it. Although it is essential to hear service users expressing their desire to change, confidence in their ability to achieve it still needs to be built. The person needs to be able to voice for themselves their own strengths and ability to make the desired change. This is much more effective than simply saying something like: *'I believe you can do it.'*

How you could do this

It is important to show confidence in the person's ability to change, and you can do this through making reflective statements which are positive. You might say something like:

'Earlier you spoke about how you successfully completed an NVQ. What skills did you use to help you achieve that?'

'You have explained to me how you compère a charity event every month in the village hall, regularly organise family get-togethers and mentor a teenage football team. It seems to me you have good communication skills to be able to do that.'

Other tactics you can use to help build confidence in ability include the following.

 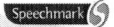

1 Use a 'Confidence in ability to change' scale, as shown in Strategy 11: 'Using a motivational balance sheet'. If the person marks a 4 on the scale, ask: *'Where would you need to be on the scale to feel confident that you would succeed in changing?'* The person might choose an 8. This can then be followed up with: *'What would need to happen for you to move up to an 8?'* This can then be explored. Alternatively, use small steps. For example: *'What would need to happen for you move up to a 5?'* This can be followed by: *'What else would need to happen to move to a 6?'* And so on.

2 Identify skills the person uses every day, or has done in the past, which would help them cope with making the change. You can use a simple form to do this, as shown in Figure 8. Guide the person to identify skills in their personal life, daily living, social life, hobbies, interests and employment.

Skills to help me change
Skills I use every day are:
Skills I have used in the past are:
Skills I can use to help me change are:

Figure 8 'Skills to help me change' form

3 Help the person identify people who will support and help them make changes. These people will include relations, friends, professionals and others they might approach for support. They can be listed on a simple chart, as suggested in Figure 9. Ensure that the person includes people who have helped them before, are in a position to help them now, and will be happy if they do change, believing they can do it.

PEOPLE WHO WILL HELP ME	
Type of people	**How they will help**
Relations	
Friends	
Professionals	
Others	

Figure 9 'People who will help me' chart

4 Explore what the person sees as barriers to their being able to change. Using the form shown in Figure 10, tease out barriers which are

- **internal**: thoughts (what others might think), fears (what the person feels they will lose if they change, such as friendships), and so on

- **external**: physical, practical, people who might not be helpful.

Invite the person to imagine that they have succeeded in changing and are looking back. What would they think about and see as solutions to these barriers?

LOOKING AT BARRIERS		
Barriers	**What I think about these barriers looking back after changing is:**	**What I could do to overcome these barriers is:**
Internal	Internal	Internal
External	External	External

Figure 10 'Looking at barriers' form

5 Ask the person to look back on times in the past when they have dealt with change. This could include the change from being a child to a teenager and then to an adult, moving from one school or job to another, leaving home, getting married or moving in with a partner, moving house to a different area, becoming a team leader or manager, training to get a qualification or take part in a competition, saving up to go on holiday or buying something, and so on.

We all go through and have to deal with many changes. Use the form in Figure 11 to help the person identify changes in the past, the strengths they used and can use again now. Examples of those strengths might be: determination, good time-keeping, good social skills, ability to see things through, enjoyment of the challenge, ability to make friends easily, coping with change a step at a time, overcoming the fear by keeping in mind what it would be like when they succeeded, and so on.

MY STRENGTHS TO HELP ME CHANGE		
Changes I have made in the past are:	Strengths I used were:	Strengths I can use now are:

Figure 11 ' My strengths to help me change' form

Comment

Using listening and reflecting skills and eliciting statements affirming abilities are essential during this process. The aim is always to draw out statements from the person that reinforce their belief in their ability to succeed.

Strategy 14: Exploring reasons for making changes

Introduction

In order for individuals to want to change, they obviously must be unhappy in some way with their current situation. The person may have been sent to you under pressure or have come voluntarily, or you have noticed their dissatisfaction with their situation and have approached them. Although the person may be unhappy in some measure with their predicament, this does not guarantee that they will make changes because they may not know how to. They may lack belief in their ability to make changes (see Strategy 13: 'Increasing belief in ability to change') or not feel sufficient dissatisfaction to motivate them into action.

Motivation may come from wanting something or wanting to avoid unease with their current situation. In reality, people are often equally motivated by fear of consequences as by wanting something (a different life, to be successful, greater status, for example). Fear of repercussions, such as having their wages docked or losing their position, might be what motivates them to get to work on time. Other motivators might include wanting to avoid bad health, or fear of loneliness or failing at something important.

Whatever motivates the person – either benefits or negative consequences – you need to find out what is important to them and encourage them to state their reasons for making changes.

How you could do this

It is important that any statements of intent to change come directly from the person. To elicit these, there is a range of questions you might try. You should then listen carefully to their answers and reflect back any statements that indicate an intention to change.

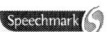

Below are some examples. You may need to rephrase some of them to suit the situation.

'How would you like things to be different in the future from the way they are now?'

'What would you change if you didn't have any constraints?'

'What would need to happen today to make this session worth while for you?'

'If you could choose a dream about how you would like your future life to be, what would you dream?'

'In how many ways does the situation create difficulties for you?'

'Could you take me through a typical week and tell me how your situation influences it?'

'In what way is this a problem for you?'

'Why is this a particular concern?'

'What makes you think you need to get to grips with this problem?'

'What are your worst fears if you don't tackle this problem?'

'How would things change for you if you decided to do something about this?'

'In what way do you hope I can help you with this problem?'

'What will happen if you do nothing?'

'What are your reasons for wanting to change?'

'What difference would it make if you did change?'

'What would you like to hear your partner/tutor/key worker say to you?'

'If you did get to grips with this problem, what would you be able to do that you can't do now?'

If the person has difficulty coming up with reasons, asking them to view their difficulty from a third-party angle can be helpful. For example:

'If your Dad were here today, what reasons would he give for why you should make some changes?'

'What do you think your brother/friend would be saying to you about this?'

'Looking at this problem from your son's point of view, what reasons might he give you?'

After the person has given their reasons, you can then reflect them back. Examples might include:

'Do I understand you correctly: you want to change because you love your children and want to make sure you don't lose your job and can provide them with a secure childhood?'

'Are saying you want to change because you want this relationship to work and are afraid that if you continue running up debts and telling him lies he will leave you?'

'I understand from what you are saying that you want to be able to manage your time better, to enable you to attend each session so you can gain this qualification and get a better job.'

'Can I make sure I understand what you are saying? You have been warned that if you don't control your angry outbursts you will be excluded from the art group. But you really enjoy the sessions and want to be able to go with the group on their outings.'

'You are saying that if you do nothing the situation will become worse. You will lose the support of your partner and friends, your health will deteriorate and you will become even more depressed.'

'You are telling me your partner would be very pleased if you did something about this. He would support and encourage you and tell you how proud he is of what you are doing. Is that correct?'

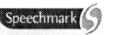

Comment

Most of these reflections naturally lead on to other techniques, such as those in Strategy 13: 'Increasing belief in ability to change' and in the 'Importance of change' and the 'Confidence in ability' scales in Strategy 11: 'Using a motivational balance sheet', as appropriate. This, in turn, prepares the person for the next stage of setting goals and planning how they will make the changes.

The person is more likely to be motivated to succeed in making the changes when these statements are made by them and reinforced in this way. It ensures that they have control of the problem or difficulty and are not giving it to you to solve.

Strategy 15: Using paradoxical statements

Introduction

This is a tactic which should be used only as a last resort and possibly with individuals who argue against any change or might want to prove that you are wrong. The process involves you amplifying negative statements made by the person in an attempt to get them to argue against you about the importance of making changes. For example, *'You have been trying to control your eating habits for the past month, perhaps now is not the right time to make changes.'* The statements are intended to be perceived by the person as an unexpected contradiction, invoking them to respond by saying they *do* want to change. This can then lead to a conversation identifying the reasons why there is little or no progress. The risk is that the person might agree with your paradoxical statement. It is a tactic that is safest used after the person has established that they do want to change, but there is no progress beyond this.

How you could do this

You need to listen to what the person is saying and amplify and reflect the statements back in a paradoxical way. The person may be arguing against making changes, how they cannot do it and it is all hopeless. They may even be deliberately trying to provoke or divert you. You must respond in a calm and sincere manner. Any sign of exasperation, impatience or sarcasm will lead to failure. Examples of statements include:

'You say you enjoy and want to stay in the music group and yet you continue to be disruptive. Perhaps now is not the right time for you to be in the group?'

'You do seem to have a lot going on at present: trying to cope with a new job, your son having an accident, your mother needing support and your husband away two or three days each week. I can't help wondering if this is the right time to be making these changes?'

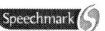

'We have discussed a number of options you could take for making changes. I have the impression that they lack appeal for you and that you might be quite happy with things as they are. In which case, might it be better for you to continue exactly as you are?'

'I'm wondering if you are ready to tackle this problem at the moment. Maybe you are not motivated enough?'

'We have discussed the reasons for you to make changes as well as those for you to stay the same. It appears to me that your reasons for staying the same still outweigh your reasons to change. Could it be that you really want things to remain as they are?'

'From what you are saying, it is clearly going to be hard for you to make these changes. Maybe you couldn't do it if you tried?'

'Making changes at this time might be too difficult for you.'

'I don't know if you are ready to handle these changes at present.'

Comment

If the process results in self-motivation statements, it is working. If the person does not respond immediately by arguing for change, suggest that they think about what has been said and arrange to see them again at a later date. However, do be aware that this tactic does not always work, and the person may decide that they do not want to change. If this is the case, discuss with them the reasons for this; it might also be appropriate to suggest that you see them at a later date to explore any further developments in their thinking about making changes.

Strategy 16: Normalising situations

Introduction

'Normalising' is a method of communicating to individuals that it is not unusual to have difficulties when making changes. Talking about their concerns as if they are common – rather than exceptional – life events can help to reduce their anxieties. It reassures them that they are not alone in feeling ambivalent or crazy or that they are an outsider, or in feeling embarrassed or thinking they are doomed. When they understand that others have similar experiences and these can be described in normal everyday terms, they feel more at ease and able to discuss their problems. Normalising is the opposite of catastrophising and making something appear dramatic. It is not intended to make the person feel comfortable with not making changes, but to show that it is normal to experience difficulty.

How you could do this

Normalising is responding to information in a matter-of-fact manner. To aid this you can also discuss other situations, similar to the one presented. This helps the person to understand that their situation is not unique and is not unusual or unacceptable to others. This does not mean you ignore or dismiss issues which the person finds worrying and important. But it does mean acknowledging their concern or worry without expressing their sense of anxiety or stress about it. The following examples show how you might do this.

Service user:	*'I have made several attempts to reduce my weight but nothing seems to work.'*
Worker:	*'Many people find this difficult. They often say they have made a number of attempts. What methods have you tried?'*
Service user:	*'The whole situation gets me down. I feel depressed and have even thought of committing suicide.'*
Worker:	*'It's not unusual for people to think like that. What you are doing is difficult. Did you seriously think of suicide or was it one of those thoughts we all get from time to time when we are feeling overwhelmed?'*
Service user:	*'When I go out, I keep thinking people are looking at me.'*
Worker:	*'I can see that is worrying you. It is a concern that many people have. Can we spend a few minutes talking about it?'*
Service user:	*'I felt foolish and got embarrassed. Then I forgot what to say.'*
Worker:	*'Most people feel like that at first. What helped you cope with the situation?'*
Service user:	*'Condoms. I don't usually use them.'*
Worker:	*'Some people say sex is better when they use them. Others that they get in the way or they feel silly putting them on. What's your experience?'*

Comment

Making statements like these enables the person to feel they are not alone with their problem. It reduces it to normality and helps them feel more at ease talking about it. It also diminishes any feelings they have of being out of step with normal or expected behaviour and gives them permission to elaborate on their experiences.

Strategy 17: Encouraging 'success' talk

Introduction

Enabling individuals to talk about 'successful' behaviour encourages them to engage in that behaviour. Simulating doing something is similar to performing it. This means that when you describe yourself doing something in detail, you increase the chances of actually doing it. Talking about success and being able to picture it also helps to build confidence in being able to succeed.

How you could do this

Here are some example questions to help lead into 'success' talk.

'What would you like to achieve?'

'What would improve for you if you did overcome this problem?'

'What would be different for you if you were more assertive?'

'What would be the best outcome for you?'

'Can you describe to me how you would like things to be?'

'What are you doing now that you would like to do more of?'

'Tell me, what would you like to be doing one year from today?'

'How have you coped with this in the past? What would happen if you did that now?'

Follow the replies with other statements which help the person to give full details. Remember to use positive body language as you do so. Examples of such statements include:

'What else would be different?'

 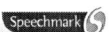

'What would that mean to you?'

'How would you feel when that happened?'

'Tell me more.'

If, before you are able to ask any of the above questions, the person starts by describing a situation that appears to be negative, ask them how they would like to deal with the situation in the future. For example:

Worker:	*'I know you find these situations difficult to cope with. Tell me, though, how you would like to deal with Margery trying to dominate the conversation and not listening to what you have to say. You might not be able to do it, but how would you like to respond?'*
Service user:	*'It's not easy. I wouldn't want to offend her. I suppose I would tell her that I value what she has to say, but I would like her to stop talking for a moment, listen to what I have to say and take my opinions into account.'*

The worker can now repeat this back and move forwards by enabling the person to state that this is what she wants to do, building confidence and action planning as appropriate. In the above case, it may be helpful to role-play the situation, with the worker taking the part of Margery.

Comment

The fact that the person has identified the difficulty, envisaged her own solution, said it aloud in her own words and role-played carrying it out will increase the chances of success. This is a tactic which can be useful at all stages of the motivation process.

Strategy 18: Using reflective listening skills to roll with resistance

Introduction

Resistance can be subtle. Service users may challenge you in a direct and argumentative way or in a subtle manner. This might include such statements as:

'There's no point in changing now.'

'Stopping would be too hard.'

'I don't understand why my son and you are so bothered about this. It's my life and I can do what I want.'

'I can't stand people telling me what to do.'

'I suppose you're going to tell me you won't let me go on the outing.'

In motivational interviewing, the process is to recognise this as a sign of ambivalence and avoid arguing about the issue. This process – called rolling with resistance – has the effect of reducing, rather than increasing, resistance.

How you could do this

Below are described a few ways in which you could approach this.

Shift the focus

Sometimes it is easier to acknowledge and go round the barrier by emphasising personal choice rather than to go head on into it.
For example:

'You are correct. Stopping will be difficult. You may choose not to. We are just going to discuss the issue. It's up to you to decide what you want to do.'

 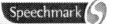

'I've no intention of telling you what to do. That's up to you. You will have to make that decision yourself.'

'You said you want to go on the outing. My intention is to explore what you can do to enable that to happen. You decide what you will do.'

Reframe the meaning

Reframing has been defined as 'the art of attributing different meaning to behaviour so the behaviour will be seen differently' (Constantine *et al*, 1984, p313). To do this, you acknowledge the truth in the person's statement. This is achieved by shifting their perspective by modifying the meaning behind their behaviour. The aim is to enable them to view and approach the situation differently. It is a way to introduce new ideas without being confrontational.

To do this, you need to reframe negative elements in a positive way. Some examples are shown below.

Service user:	*'I'm hopeless at interviews.'*
Worker:	*'You've pinpointed what you need to work on from past experience. That's a good place to start.'*
Service user:	*'I can't stop myself speaking out if I think something is wrong. It gets me into terrible arguments and, yes, I upset people. Everyone dislikes me. They think I'm out to make trouble when I just want to do a good job.'*
Worker:	*'It sounds like you have some leadership qualities. What would happen if you were able to speak up without getting into arguments and upsetting people?'*

Service user:	'I've tried a number of times but nothing works!'
Worker:	'Sounds like you've been trying hard and experiencing a lot of frustration. It's good that you have been exploring possibilities and finding out what works and doesn't work for you. Tell me what you've tried so far.'
Service user:	'I've got to work long hours to give my family everything they want.'
Worker:	'That shows great concern and dedication. You are doing your best to make them happy. How do you imagine they might see it?'

Use straight reflections

To do this, rephrase or repeat what the person has said. This lets them know that you have heard and you are not going to argue with them.

Service user:	'I can't stop smoking. It helps me relax and most of my friends smoke.'
Worker:	'You feel giving up smoking will be nearly impossible because you find it relaxing and most of your friends smoke.'
Service user:	'Yeah, that's it. I know I should but there it is.'
Worker:	'Would you think differently if neither of these were an issue?'

Amplify reflections

This is similar to using straight reflections. Here you exaggerate the reflection to the point where the person disagrees with it. Do be careful, though, not to overdo this or the person may feel patronised or that you are being sarcastic, and may respond with anger.

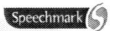

Service user:	*'I argue with my tutor because it gets me respect from my mates.'*
Worker:	*'I see. You keep interrupting and arguing with the tutor because it's the only way you feel you can earn respect from others in the class.'*
Service user:	*'No. But it's one way of showing I'm there and won't be ignored.'*

Double-sided reflections

This tactic requires you to reflect the current statement which shows resistance and a previous contradictory statement the person has made.

Service user:	*'I can't keep to a diet. Everybody else eats what they like. I don't want to be any different.'*
Worker:	*'You don't want to have to keep to a diet but, at the same time, you're concerned about the effect eating what you like has on your health. Is that correct?'*
Service user:	*'Yes. I feel pulled between the two. When I'm on my own it's OK, but when I'm with other people I feel left out.'*

Avoid being led astray

Sometimes, service users will hint or give the impression that they are not giving important information or are withholding it and avoid direct discussion about it. You may find yourself wondering what it might be, how significant it is, and whether you should pursue it. If you do pursue it, the person uses different tactics to avoid confronting the issue, with the result that nothing is achieved.

If you find that this is happening, you need to explore whether the person has any fears about exposing the information. This could include issues of trust, confidentiality, talking about something the person considers shocking, thinking you will be shocked, gender, embarrassment, or fear of consequences. A discussion around these issues and time spent addressing any fears usually results in the difficulty coming out into the open.

If it is not revealed, and the person continues to give signals, but keeps leading you along false trails, it is likely that they are using it as a method of diverting you, to avoid facing the real problem, and to use up time. In these instances, avoid chasing the issue. Use a paradoxical approach. Do this by saying something like:

'I sense there's something you want to say but feel unsure about it. I'm aware how hard it is to talk about sensitive matters and there are some things you might not want to tell me. So, it might be best if we don't discuss this particular issue now. When you feel ready, we can come back to whatever it is that's worrying you. In the meantime, perhaps we can talk about the things you do feel comfortable about telling me.'

This moves the conversation on. If the person later returns to the same avoidance tactic, repeat the process and give assurance that when they are ready to talk about the matter, you will listen. The message will soon be picked up that you are not prepared to be led along false trails. This usually results in either the details being revealed eventually or the matter not being mentioned again. Generally, if it is something important, it will crop up more than once in the conversation. If it does not, it is likely that you were being diverted.

Comment

When the person starts arguing against change, they talk themselves out of making any changes and fortify their resistance. Directly opposing resistance will have the same result. Rolling with resistance is a method of avoiding this happening and preventing a breakdown in your communication with the person. Which method you use will depend on your judgement of what will work best in any particular situation.

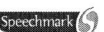

Strategy 19: Prompting talk about change

Introduction

An important part of motivating people is prompting them to talk about making changes and then reinforcing the positive aspects discussed. This applies to discussions about Desire, Ability, Reason, Need and Commitment to change (DARN-C for short). The fact is that when someone talks about these aspects of change, and what is said is generated from within themselves, they are much more likely to be motivated than if someone else makes suggestions to them.

You are probably aware of this from your own experience. You might have struggled with a problem for some time and then talked it through with a friend, family member or colleague. Defining and stating the problem and solution aloud, and then having this reinforced by your friend, probably convinced you to go ahead with your plan.

To enable this to happen for the service user, you need to listen carefully for the opportunity to encourage talk about change.

How you could do this

Ask evocative questions. Make these open-ended or prompting statements. Some of them may be to increase the person's anxiety or confirm any aspect of DARN-C. Some examples are:

'Can you explain why you would want to do this?' (Desire)

'Have you thought about how you might go about this?' (Ability)

'Share with me what are your reasons for doing this?' (Reasons)

'How important is it for you to succeed with this change?' (Need)

'Have you made up your mind what you're going to do?' (Commitment)

To increase the person's concern about the current situation, or to unbalance what seems an equal argument in the person's mind, emphasise the negative side of their behaviour:

'Tell me, what would your boyfriend say worries him the most?'

'You've told me what you enjoy about ... What's the down side to it?'

'You mentioned earlier about the effect this is having on your wife. Can you tell me a bit more about that?'

Look back. Ask about a time in the past before the current problems emerged:

'Describe to me a time in the past when things were better.'

'You said this started about a year ago. What was different before that?'

'You told me that there was a period, nearly a year, when you didn't get into trouble. What was different then?'

Be aware that there is a risk with questions about the past. The person will often say they do not remember a time when things were different. If they do, you will have to move on quickly to a different approach.

Look forward. Enquire about the future:

'Tell me, what do you think will happen if you continue as you are at present?'

'Describe for me what would you like life to be like for you five years from now?'

'If you were successful in making the changes you want, what would be different?'

Use goals and values. Having established what goals and values are important to the person, use those to check how current behaviour fits with them, for example as follows.

 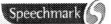

'Earlier you said that it was very important that you support your family. How does your current behaviour help with that?'

'Help me understand how you see this behaviour helping you achieve what you want.'

'Can you see any ways in which what you're doing clashes with your ambition to gain this qualification?'

Explore worst and best case scenarios. Ask about the worst and the best things that could happen:

'If you don't do anything, what is the worst thing that could happen?'

'What is the best thing that could happen if you were to change?'

Comment

You might also choose to use a motivational balance sheet or a change scale (see Strategy 11: 'Using a motivational balance sheet'). It is a mistake to rush or jump this 'talking about change' stage. If you feel the person is moving slightly ahead of you and pulling you after them, that is good and how it should be. They should be taking the lead with you a step behind. When the person has discussed and voiced DARN-C in their own words, they are ready to move on to planning the change.

Strategy 20: Watching your language

Introduction

The techniques in this book involve the use of language to lead people we are helping into better habits of thought and action. What we say and how we say it is a major factor in disrupting resistance to change, helping people find solutions to their problems and motivating them. How we speak – and the words we use – enables the person to identify what is helpful to them and what is not.

In order to do this effectively, we need to cultivate better habits in the use of language and thought ourselves. Doing so will enable us to create more useful conversations and possibilities that make something that is abstract more real and concrete for the person we are helping. In the words of O'Hanlon and Weiner-Davis (1989, p60), 'It [language] can be used as a tool to question unhelpful realities.'

A good way to start raising your awareness and forming good habits as you carry out day-to-day tasks is to try the following suggestions, one at a time. You may already be using some of them.

How you could do this

Imply that change is constant

To allow a person to assume otherwise is likely to lead to behaviour that encourages resistance. Reminders that change is constant are particularly useful when the person appears to be stuck and is undecided. This indicates that their state of stagnation is temporary and movement in the desired direction is on the horizon. Use phrases that imply change, rather than direct statements. These will be picked up subconsciously. Here are a few examples:

'At the moment, you just want to talk about your concerns with your son.'

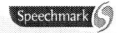

'You don't currently feel ready to discuss issues around going on the outing.'

'Right now, you feel angry and don't want to consider other options.'

'At this point, you are finding it difficult to face talking about this.'

Enable the use of metaphors

Metaphor is a figure of speech which implies a comparison. Metaphors can be simple comparisons or similes, allegories or parables. Simple metaphors make simple comparisons, such as *'He has a heart of stone'*, *'white as a sheet'* or *'light as a feather'*. Common metaphors like these become clichés. However, what they do is convey the unknown by relating it to something already known. Complex metaphors are stories with different levels of meaning. People make use of stories to convey meaning that is difficult to communicate.

Our thought processes are largely metaphorical (Lakoff & Johnson, 1980). This makes metaphor a powerful and effective device when communicating and working with service users. Below is a short example taken from a conversation in a day centre that encouraged the service user to use metaphor when she was having difficulty conveying how she felt about living on her own since her partner died in a car accident.

Worker:	*'Being on your own is like …?'*
Service user:	*'It's like being stuck in a marsh. I'm sinking and can't move. I'm yelling and reaching out and there's no one there to help me.'*
Worker:	*'Have you any thoughts about what would help you?'*
Service user:	*'Courage. I really need to stop hiding away from people.'*
Worker:	*'Tell me, if you had courage and stopped hiding away from people, what would life be like? What would you be doing?'*

This same method can be applied in different situations by placing it in a specific context. For example:

'When you're in the class, it is like …?'

'When you get angry, it is like …?'

'When things are going well, it is like …?'

'When the craving is bad, it is like …?'

'When you feel happy, it is like …?'

'Being stuck, not knowing what to do, is like …?

When the person has provided the metaphor, you can then begin to ask developmental questions. Do be careful, though, that the questions you ask are not phrased in a way that might lead the person in the direction you *think* they should go. What the person states should come from within themselves.

Sometimes, people need time to think about the metaphors, so pause and avoid rushing. Some might also find it easier to write or draw a metaphor.

Move from general to specific

Individuals often make sweeping generalisations such *as 'I'm always late',* *'I don't get any sleep', 'I can't do anything right', 'I've always been anxious'* or *'I must always be in control.'* In these instances it is helpful to guide the person to examine any evidence for their statement and to be specific. To do this, you need to be careful not to deny the person's view of things, while gently challenging and establishing a more realistic view of this type of exaggerated thinking and putting it into perspective. The following is an example of this.

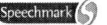

Service user:	*'I never do anything right.'*
Worker:	*'I can see why you might feel like that at the moment. Is it OK if we look at the evidence for what you are saying?'*
Service user:	*'OK.'*
Worker:	*'You told me earlier that the class went well on Monday. The tutor congratulated you on your work. You also managed to cook a meal for your mother. What else have you done this week?'*
Service user:	*'I went shopping with my sister and then we saw a film. I took the dog to the vet for his injection. I vacuumed the lounge.'*
Worker:	*'So, in fact, you are saying that most of the time you do do things right.'*
Service user:	*'Yes, I suppose I do.'*
Worker:	*'Can you tell me what went wrong on this particular occasion?'*

By reflecting inconsistencies and helping individuals challenge themselves, the aim is to allow them to draw their own conclusions. Make the approach an invitation for exploration. This helps to avoid the challenge coming across too strongly, which could be perceived as trying to put them down. Working in this way leads to less resistance than challenging someone directly.

Add to existing statements, behaviour and ideas

It is always easier to add to existing behaviour and ideas the person has than to get them to accept completely new ones. To do this, you need to find out what they are already doing and suggest they do something extra. The addition is then less likely to encounter resistance. The following are some examples.

'You come to the lounge each morning for tea. Perhaps you could stay a little longer and join in the discussion group?'

'You say you are enjoying the singing group. Have you thought what other activities you would like to do?'

'At the moment you have told only me about your difficulty. Who else might it be helpful to tell?'

'You now feel comfortable staying in the group for 30 minutes. How do you feel about extending that to 45 minutes?'

'When you come down to breakfast each morning, could you bring any dirty laundry with you and put it in the laundry basket, please?'

Embed suggestions

This is a way of indirectly putting an idea into a service user's mind. The person does not feel that it is being imposed on them or that they are being directed. Consequently, it is not thought of as threatening and they give it serious consideration. Sometimes, it can later emerge as the service user's own idea. You would only do this in order to direct the person in a way which benefits them and fits with their values, beliefs and goals and not with your own view of what you think is best for them. The suggestion should always be positive and move them in the direction they want to go.

Many of the techniques in this book use embedded suggestions. These are usually included as part of a reflection. There are some examples overleaf. Note that the worker responses also indicate that the current state is not permanent.

 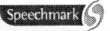

Service user:	'I'm too frightened to stand up to him.'
Worker:	'At the moment you feel frightened of John. It's hard for you to imagine yourself saying "No".'

Service user:	'I get so impatient and angry. It's like he's doing it to upset me. I know it's because of his dementia. But I still yell at him and then feel terrible afterwards. I can't stop myself.'
Worker:	'Right now you're struggling to see how you can handle these situations differently and avoid your anger building to the point where it's out of control.'

Service user:	'I just can't see a way forward. Whatever I do will be wrong.'
Worker:	'Currently, you're caught in a quandary and are searching for a way to weigh up the reasons "for" and "against" what you want to do.'

Service user:	'I can't do interviews. I'm so nervous I can't think. My mind goes blank. I can't concentrate or answer the questions. My mouth dries up and I get soaked in sweat. There's no point in going.'
Worker:	'Right now you find interviews extremely difficult and are looking to find a way to help you stay calm and focus on and answer any questions you are asked.'

Use the word 'if' with care

When working with people you are aiming to motivate to change their behaviour, it is necessary, as mentioned above, to imply that change is constant. This indicates your belief in the person's ability to make the change. If you speak in terms of 'if' when discussing that behaviour, you are sending a message that is in conflict with that belief. There is an underlying supposition that the service user may not change; thus, the word may contribute to resistance. This is easily remedied by replacing 'if' with words or phrases that do imply change. For example:

'If you try this out, you'll find that ...' becomes *'When you try this out, you'll find that ...'*

'If you make progress in the assertiveness skills group, your confidence will grow' becomes *'As you make progress in the assertiveness skills group, you'll find that your confidence grows.'*

'If you adapt to the new situation you can ...' becomes *'While adapting to the new situation you can ...'*

Although it is not helpful to use 'if' when referring to future desirable actions, when you apply it while discussing current undesirable behaviour, it has the opposite effect. It suggests that this behaviour does not have to be permanent. For example:

'If you continue to disrupt the class, tell me what you think will happen.'

'What will be the effect on your health if you don't change your eating habits?'

'If you refuse to comply with the safety procedures, what is the likely outcome?'

Avoid 'Yes, but ...'

This is an expression which starts by appearing to agree, but actually indicates disagreement and resistance: *'Yes, but I don't have time to ...'* It frequently leads to a discussion that is a dispute about who is right. It is, in fact, a statement which says *'No'*.

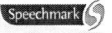

Guard against this type of response by waiting for a direct request for information or advice, or ask for permission first and then seem reluctant. When you present it, do so in a way that allows the person to judge how it might be applicable to them:

'I've got an idea, but I'm not sure it would be right for you.'

'I wouldn't want you to think I'm telling you what to do. I can make a few suggestions, but you need to decide whether they would work for you.'

'Someone else I know tried ... Would that work for you?'

If you find you are using the phrase *'Yes, but if you don't do something about this ...'*, the discussion again ends up in a dispute with the person showing resentment that you are trying to force them into action. In these instances, try replacing the *'Yes, but ...'* with *'Yes, and ...'*. This normally leads the conversation into a more useful and positive direction and improves cooperation:

'Yes, and would this be an opportunity to do ...?'

'Yes, and you also said you wanted ...'

'Yes, and does that mean ...?'

Be aware of the effect of using 'we'

'We' is another word that can work in a negative way, particularly with service users who are uncooperative or resistant to change. Normally, the word is used in a way that is intended to be supportive, and indeed can be, if the person is highly motivated. However, when you use it with someone who has a problem, is uncooperative or is resistant to change, you are inviting them to pass on the responsibility for both the problem and its resolution to you. You are going to provide a miracle solution with little or no effort from them and you will get the blame when it does not work. Doing this also contributes to making the person dependent.

The use of 'we' can also lead into prolonged, difficult discussions in which you are attempting to give back to the service user the responsibility for resolving the problem, making the changes or taking action.

To avoid the service user assuming a passive role, and disempowering them, instead of making statements such as *'We will work on this'*, try something like *'I will support you while you work through this.'* Two other examples are:

Instead of *'Let's see what we can do about this'*, try *'Would you like to discuss some of your ideas for dealing with this?'*

Instead of *'I wonder what we can do about this?'*, try *'Have you thought about what you would like to do about this?'*

The aim is to keep the responsibility for both the problem and its resolution where it belongs – with the individual. In this way you also guard against any erosion of their independence.

Focus attention by using names

After greeting someone, it is amazing how quickly we replace their name with 'you' for the remainder of the conversation. Yet, it is a fact that when we hear our own name mentioned, we immediately tune in and pay particular attention to what is being said. This can be used in a positive way to increase attention to the point you are making. The person's name can be dropped into a statement at the beginning, middle or end. The effect can be accentuated by pausing briefly after using the name. Here are a few examples:

'Peter, tell me what you feel are the advantages of ...'

'As you think ahead and see yourself gaining confidence, Jean, describe how ...'

'It's OK to feel angry when something like this happens. It's a normal reaction, Richard.'

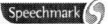

Dropping in someone's name in this way from time to time, as well as having the effect of focusing attention more closely on what is being said, also gives the service user the impression that you are giving them close personal attention.

Check for distorted thinking

Distortions happen when we make an assumption about what someone is feeling, how they might react, or what they want to do without first checking this. By making assumptions about what the person is thinking, we become 'mind readers'. Often, we get it wrong and the end result is a loss of rapport with the person we are trying to help.

You know that distortions are in play and you are making assumptions when you catch yourself thinking or saying things such as:

'I know what you mean.'

'You must be so embarrassed.'

'You must feel very hurt.'

'You must feel proud.'

You may not know what the person is thinking or feeling at all, but are assuming something quite different. In these instances, ask yourself *'How do I know this?'* and check exactly what the other person *is* feeling:

'How did you feel about that?'

'What is your understanding about ...?'

Comment

Some of the language uses discussed here may seem minor, but they do provide a greatly increased benefit, particularly when you are working with service users who are considered uncooperative or resistant to making changes that would benefit them.

Strategy 21: Approaching difficult topics

Introduction

There is a wide range of difficult topics in care, health and educational settings. These can vary from hygiene issues to behaviour that puts health at risk, is disruptive to others or is interfering with people's progress towards achieving goals. The person may or may not be aware of their problem. Either way, the subject may be a difficult one that is likely to encounter resistance. In these cases, once the issue has been broached, you will need to rely heavily on your active listening skills to bring the relationship back into harmony and resolve the matter.

How you could do this

Having ensured that you are approaching the person in a suitable environment that enables them to feel comfortable, safe and, if necessary, supported, it is helpful to open with a statement that contains the following three elements.

A direct statement of your concerns. Avoid using the word 'problem' when doing this as it can immediately prompt a defensive and resistant attitude. You may also come across as being judgemental. It may be regarded as a problem for you or others, but not by the person himself or herself. Instead, use words such as 'concern', 'issue', 'matter' or 'regarding ...'. Give the issue some thought beforehand and ensure that the statement is made without being judgemental. Incorporate, where possible and as appropriate, previous disclosures about commitments or the issue at hand.

A comment about the person's responsibility for choice and change. This puts the ball firmly in their court and indicates that you are not telling them what to do. It is their choice.

A question at the end of your statement asking for their view on the subject. The person may or may not be motivated to be open and honest about the situation. The task is to make them feel safe enough to be able to explore and resolve it. Do this by adapting an attitude of concern about the person's welfare, exploring and trying to understand and resolve the matter, rather than being confrontational and trying to prove that they are in the wrong. Information gathered from them in this way will help you suggest ideas that will be in line with their needs and desires and contribute to a resolution.

It may also be useful for you to have worked out an agenda for yourself that will guide and help you focus the session. However, do not treat this as a rigid plan. Be open to alterations and changes of direction. It can also be helpful to use 'normalising' comments, to communicate to the person that their situation is not uncommon and make it easier for them to talk about the subject (see Strategy 16: 'Normalising situations').

Here is an example, using the three-stage approach discussed above:

> 'It's not unusual for students to experience difficulties at this stage of their course. I'm concerned that the tutor had to send you home yesterday after lunch because you had been drinking and kept falling asleep in class. My worry is that this puts you in danger of returning to your old drinking habits and it also puts your placement on the course at risk. When we last spoke, you said your top priority was to complete the course and gain your qualification so you could get a job. You also said that your partner had threatened to leave you if you didn't sort yourself out and you didn't want that to happen. What you choose to do, of course, is up to you. What do you think about these concerns?'

Comment

Workers in care, educational or health environments are in positions in which they should voice and address concerns about their students' or service users' health or decisions which are harmful. This needs to be done in a manner which avoids being judgemental or arguing with them. Instead, invite the person to consider information that may change their decision. This is different from approving or condoning any harmful behaviour.

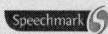

SECTION 3

Supporting people when they plan the change (Determination)

The person is ready to change and needs to prepare and plan how to go about doing so. Sometimes people will want to rush ahead without adequate planning. Skimping on this stage and leaping into action can increase the chances of failure or inadequate change. During the process of planning, the person will decide on the specific steps they will take to solve the problem. This will help them build confidence and increase their belief in their ability to change.

The process now involves the person setting goals, choosing from options to achieve those goals, exploring the skills needed to achieve them, deciding on a plan, and providing a verbal statement of commitment.

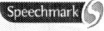

Strategy 22: Making sure the person is ready to change

Introduction

Timing is paramount when spotting the right moment to move on to begin talking about setting goals and planning any changes to be made. If you move on too soon, you increase the risk of problems cropping up later in the process and the person relapsing. Sometimes you may find that, when the person comes to you, they have already decided that they want to make changes, but are at a loss as to how to go about doing so.
To make sure the person is ready and has the best chance of success, you need to spot when, or if, they are ready to start planning the change.

How you could do this

Indications that the person is not yet ready to change will be apparent if they continue to:

- put up arguments against changing

- blame others

- minimise the problem

- talk, or talk more, about the problem.

In these instances, you will need to focus on strengthening the importance of changing and building their confidence.

Signs that they are ready to start talking about setting goals and planning the change include the following.

- Indications that they are feeling a sense of loss and resignation. They are deciding to give up something they had positive as well as negative thoughts about, so this is natural. Signs of resignation show that they are close to making, or are ready to make, the decision to change.

- They may seem more calm and peaceful. The arguments in their mind have been resolved to their satisfaction, they feel that they want to make the change, and they have enough confidence in their ability to do so.

- They start discussing the advantages of change. They have persuaded themselves that it is right for them and are focusing on what they will gain.

- They begin to visualise and discuss difficulties they would have to overcome if they made the change. They are not using this as an argument against changing, but imagining what change would be like and how they would cope.

- They make positive expressions of hope for the future and you pick up a sense of their readiness to move on.

Comment

If the person has come to you and states that they are ready to change, and they want to rush ahead, you will still need to check out their Desire, Ability, Reasons, Need and Commitment to change (DARN-C) (see Strategy 19:'Prompting talk about change'). If you feel confident that the person is ready to move on, follow the process in Strategy 23: 'Negotiating goals'.

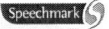

Strategy 23: Negotiating goals

Introduction

A good way to progress from discussing change to talking about setting goals is to summarise the reasons for change. The summary should contain:

- the person's own perception of the problem behaviour, incorporating the disadvantages if nothing changes

- a recognition of anything that still appeals about the old behaviour

- an outline of any objective evidence that is important

- an emphatic summation of their stated intention and confidence to make the change

- your own assessment of the situation and confidence in the person's ability to succeed.

This sums up the situation, clarifies and reinforces the person's stated reasons for making changes, and acknowledges any remaining hesitations. There may not be total resolution of all issues, but there should be sufficient commitment and confidence to start talking about setting goals.

How you could do this

Any goals should be the choice of the person setting them. Any attempt to impose or force what you think should be their goals will usually meet with resistance. You can make suggestions if the person is struggling, but only after asking for permission to do so.

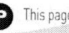

All goals should be **SMART**, that is:

Specific. General goals tend to be vague. Specific goals are simple and state what the person wants to happen. Instead of a general goal to lose weight and be healthier, they set a specific goal to lose 10 pounds or walk five miles on five days each week. This incorporates what they are going to do, and why and how they are going to do it, stated in a positive way. If a goal is a behavioural one, perhaps to respond to someone in an assertive way, then the circumstances in which that behaviour will be used can be incorporated into the goal statement.

Measurable. This enables progress to be monitored. A good question to ask to ensure a measurable goal is: *'How will you know when you have achieved your goal?'* An example answer might be: *'I will be able to stay in the art room with the others and remain focused for the whole session.'*

Appealing. Goals need to fit with personal values and other ambitions to ensure that they are inspiring.

Realistic. A goal needs to stretch the person, but it must be realistic. The person has to feel reasonably confident that they can achieve it. If it is too difficult, or they have not yet acquired the skills to achieve it, they will become despondent and give up. This often means breaking down the goals into small, but achievable, steps or milestones.

Time limited. Another good question to ask is: *'By when do you want to have achieved this goal?'* This sets a time span within which the goal or step is to be achieved.

Goals should also be framed in a positive way: to achieve something that is wanted rather than something that is not wanted. For example: *'I want to improve my relationship with my classmates by controlling my temper'*, rather than *'I don't want to keep losing my temper with my classmates.'*

 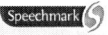

If the person wants to set goals which are unrealistic then, rather than arguing or trying to impose different goals, try questioning and reflecting inconsistencies. In this way, you can nurture in them a more realistic viewpoint and enable them to decide any necessary adjustments for themselves.

To start the process of setting goals, you will need to ask a key question, such as:

'What do you want to do?'

'What do you think you should do next?'

'What do you see as your options?'

'It sounds as though you don't want things to stay as they are. What do you think you will do now?'

'Where might you go from here?'

'Where does this leave you?'

'Have you thought about what you want to do now?'

You will need to use the same skills as you did when arousing interest and encouraging change – that is, listening, observing, reflecting meaning and clarifying (see Strategy 7: 'Using active listening skills'). The same type of questions will help you enable the person to set goals that they can realistically achieve. As already mentioned, avoid any temptation to allow your own ideas of what these should be to force their decision, or to set goals for them. If you do, these are unlikely to motivate or, indeed, to be achieved at all. The person will resist or give up at the first hurdle. The goals must be stated by and owned by the person. Again, as mentioned above, you can, of course, suggest additional goals, but only after asking permission to do so. Asking permission and putting forward your suggestions *only* as suggestions will emphasise the person's own control over the goal they end up setting for themselves.

If the goals the person wants to set seem unrealistic, check this by asking them to rate their confidence in being able to achieve them; also, check points such as the time frame that has been set. You may also need to query whether the goals are in line with the person's values and beliefs by asking: *'How does this fit with your earlier statement that ...?'* If an action seems incongruent, you can ask them to consider what they think the consequences of taking that particular action will be.

Sometimes, individuals set more than one goal. In this instance, you may need to ask them to prioritise which they will tackle first, to avoid them taking on too much and risking not achieving any of them. Success in achieving one goal will build confidence for taking on others.

Finally, you will need to ask: *'How will you know when you have achieved this goal?'* Invite the person to state what they will be doing, how they will feel and what others around them will think. The answers are the measure by which the person will know whether they have achieved their goal and by which to judge their success. Asking this question will also be useful in helping the person to set stages along the way to help monitor progress.

Comment

It is important that the goals set are realistic and the person feels reasonably confident in their ability to achieve them. If they are not then you will need to ask: *'What would need to happen to make you feel confident you could do this?'* The way in which the person answers can then be used to create stepping stones or stages on the way to achieving their goal.

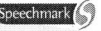

Strategy 24: Planning the change

Introduction

Once clear goals have been set, the next stage is to help the person plan how they will attain them. There are many ways in which these goals can be achieved. Different methods work for different people and, as a consequence, many options need to be explored. Only the individuals themselves know what will work best for them. They may also be feeling overwhelmed and unsure about what to do first. The aim at this point is to draw out as many options as possible, no matter how insignificant they seem, and then ask the person you are working with to select steps that suit them personally.

How you could do this

The process can be started by asking: *'How do you think you will go about doing this?'*, *'What is the first step you could take?'*, *'Have you thought about what you can do to achieve this goal?'* or *'What do you need to do to achieve this?'* Such questions open up discussion about the steps that need to be taken. The person may either have lots of ideas or be at a loss and want you to provide the plan. Be careful not to become directive. Ask permission before offering ideas or suggestions, and frame any suggestion along the lines of: *'Other people have tried ... and found that worked. What do you think?'*

As the person comes up with ideas, you can add further suggestions. Do not be afraid of including ideas that seem a bit extreme. The person will choose what is best for them. If they start making statements such as: *'That won't work, I don't have the skills'*, *'I couldn't do that because I don't have any transport'* or *'I'm not confident enough to do that'*, ask **'What if ...?'** questions:

'*What if* you attended a short course to acquire the skills?'

'*What if* transport was available?'

'*What if* you were able to build enough confidence?'

'*What if* someone helped you with that?'

These types of question can often lead into a discussion that finds solutions to obstacles or explores other options from which to choose. It may be helpful to write down all the possibilities. These can be summarised and choices made. The advantages and disadvantages of different steps can be examined.

If the person likes to see things visually, you can help them create a drawing such as a mind map to show the options, as illustrated in the example in Figure 12.

My goal is:

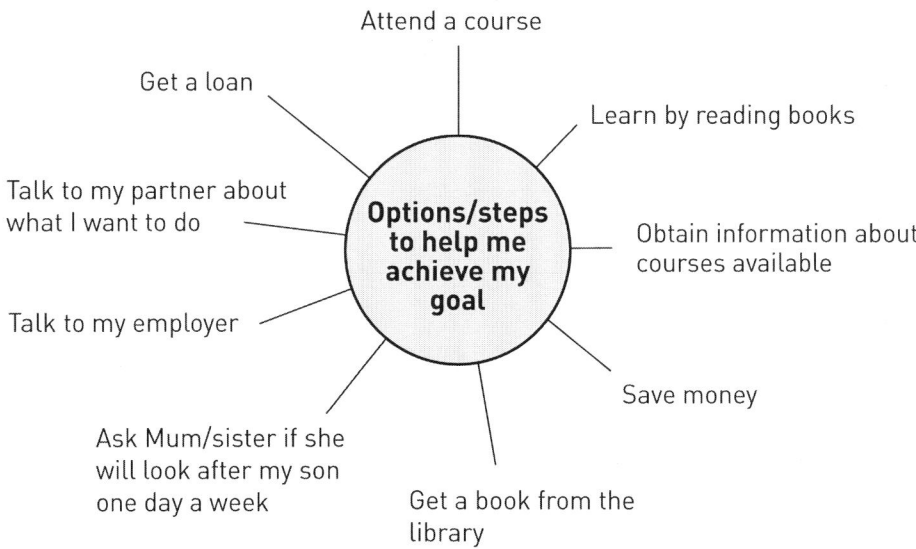

Figure 12 Using a mind map to write down options or steps

After all the ideas have been written down, choices can be made and then put into step-by-step order. Do keep in mind that the decision about which choices and steps are selected remains with the person. They need to own the plan. What seems to be the best option to you may not appeal to someone else. You should act only as a guide, gently exploring unrealistic thinking or parts of the plan which seem unworkable, or by helping the person to determine what will work best for them.

Remember to ensure the person includes in the plan their ideas about how they will record progress, and from whom, and how, they will get help if they run into difficulties. They should also include how they will make sure they complete each step. They may like to share the plan with a partner or friend who will support them. This can help ensure they carry out the actions and can add to their sense of commitment.

Once the options have been explored and the steps identified, it is usually helpful to ask the person to summarise or outline the plan. You can do this by asking: *'Just so I'm clear, what's your understanding of what you are going to do?'* Verbalising the things they are going to do reinforces the person's ownership of the plan. It is much better to put the question in this way rather than asking something like: *'Are you clear about what you are going to do?'* This can be answered with a *'Yes'* or a *'No'* – most likely *'Yes'*, even if the person is *not* clear.

Some steps may need to be broken down into smaller actions to be taken one at a time. It may be helpful for some people to write down the plan and number each action to be taken. This can be done either in the form of a simple list of steps and actions or drawn in a more visual way. For an example, see Figure 13.

Writing down (or drawing) the plan in this way also provides the person with a reminder, which they can consult as necessary, or share with other people as they wish.

GOAL ACTION PLAN		
My goal is:		
What I need to do		**When I will do it**
Step 1:	Actions: 1 2	
Step 2:	Actions: 1 2	
Step 3:	Actions: 1 2	
Step 4:	Actions: 1 2	
Step 5:	Actions: 1 2	

Figure 13 Goal action plan

Comment

Once the plan has been completed, ask the person how confident they now feel about being able to achieve their goal. If there are substantial doubts, this may mean the plan needs to be looked at again and any areas that are creating problems resolved. Asking a question such as: *'What would need to happen to make you feel confident?'* will highlight what needs to be addressed. Frequently, this can be added to the plan as a step or action. It is helpful to remind the person that some adjustments may need to be made as they progress – this could mean adding extra actions, adjusting the time deadlines and resolving problems as they arise. Life is not always predictable and allowances need to be made for adjusting plans to accommodate this.

The person will now be ready to move on to the next stage. (See Strategy 25: 'Exploring information, skills and support needed for change' and Strategy 26: 'Obtaining a statement of commitment'.)

Strategy 25: Exploring information, skills and support needed for change

Introduction

Information, skills and support all need to be explored and incorporated into steps or actions during the process of creating a plan, to ensure that the plan succeeds. The more fully it is completed, the better. It is likely, though, however thoroughly this is done, that it will need to be revisited at some point while you are mentoring the person, when unforeseen difficulties or events arise.

How you could do this

Information. The person may need additional information which you do not have available. Acquiring this will be a step or an action in the plan. Ask questions such as: *'What information do you think you will need in order to do this?'* and *'How will you obtain those details?'* The person might need help with understanding any new information. It may also change or inform later steps that are taken. Remind them that plans need to be adaptable to any changing information, events and circumstances.

Skills. Often, it is necessary to explore skills the person has acquired in the past, to help them feel confident and able to carry out any plan. They may have many transferable skills which they have not considered. Questions such as: *'You said earlier that you often organised family get-togethers. What skills did you need to do that?'* or *'Have you ever done anything similar in the past?'* are useful to tease these out and enable the person to reassess their abilities. An example of this might be someone who stays at home to bring up their children and has not been employed for some years. Frequently, they dismiss the wide range of skills needed to manage a household and raise children – being organised; contributing to meetings about the children's welfare and education; researching information about schools, among other things; budgeting;

good communication skills, and so on. Some skills may need to be acquired or built on. Again, these actions, as necessary, can be included in the plan.

Support. People are often ignorant or unaware of support that is readily available to them. This may be from relations, friends, colleagues or community or it may be work related. They may not take it up because they feel stigmatised, embarrassed or ashamed; perhaps they do not want to be beholden to someone – their pride will not allow them to be – or they have some fears around obtaining the support. Part of the process may include examining some of their negative or mistaken assumptions and dismissive thinking about the support available. These are all things which can be explored, to enable the person to decide what is or is not acceptable to them.

Rather than thinking of other people as 'support', it is helpful to encourage individuals to think about how those others could help them make the desired changes. To do this, use questions such as: 'Who would be able to help you do this?'

Comment

All of the above points require the full use of listening, reflecting and summarising skills to highlight any incongruous thinking. Often, people will be able to foresee problems or a difficulty as a plan is formulated. If they see something as an obstacle, ask: 'How do you think you might handle this?' This enables them to retain control and leaves the way open for you to make suggestions. Do not forget to preface your suggestions with statements such as: 'May I make a suggestion?' or 'Someone else in similar circumstances tried ...'

Strategy 26: Obtaining a statement of commitment

Introduction

When a plan of action has been worked out and has been summarised, the next step is to obtain confirmation that the person is committed to going ahead with it. Sometimes the commitment is obvious and you may feel this is not necessary. However, in most cases, it is a good way of exposing any doubts that the person may have about moving forwards.

How you could do this

The easiest way to elicit a statement of commitment is to ask: *'Is this what you want to do?'* The aim is that the person responds with a positive *'Yes'*. They may respond using words such as: *'I hope ...'*, *'I will try ...'*, *'I will think about this ...'*, or there may be other indications of hesitation or doubt that are shown through body language. These signs may or may not indicate a problem, but they do need a response.

The person may lack confidence, feel they are being rushed into a decision, or be worried about something that has or has not been included in the plan. Avoid pushing them into saying *'Yes'*: they may do so because they think that is what you want to hear. If they are not ready, or something important has been missed out, the plan is likely to fail.

In these instances, it is best to rely on listening, reflecting and summarising skills. Examples of ways to open up some discussion are:

'I sense that you may not be quite ready to make this decision. What worries you most about the plan?'

'It seems like you may be feeling hurried into this decision. What would need to happen for you to feel ready?'

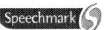

Even if nothing appears to slow progress, rather than pushing the person into saying 'Yes', you can ask them to think about it and arrange a future meeting, while emphasising their personal choice in the matter.

Comment

In the future meeting it will be important to avoid asking the person in a direct way whether they have made a decision. Instead, open with a statement such as: 'Having taken some time to think, what are your current thoughts about going ahead with the plan?' This is more likely to open up an exploratory and purposeful conversation about any problems, while leaving them free to state that they are ready to go ahead.

If there still appears to be some hesitation or lack of confidence, you can suggest a trial run of part of the plan. The person can then try a step, task or new behaviour taken from the plan to see how they feel about doing it without making a full commitment. This gives them a realistic idea of what it will be like making the changes. It can also build confidence in their ability to complete the plan.

SECTION 4

Guiding the person through planned actions (Action)

The person is now engaged in the agreed action. They may need to free themselves from previous thought patterns, control their environment, keep track of and acknowledge their progress, and reward themselves. They will need to anticipate problems, revisit some steps, change approaches, and identify and use support.

Strategy 27: The supporting role

Introduction

Depending on the circumstances, once an action plan has been formed, some individuals will be able to carry out the actions with no or little support. Others, especially when it is a longer-term plan, or the issues are more complex, will need you to provide ongoing support and guidance. This support can involve you adopting different roles during the process, which can vary between using your coaching, mentoring and counselling skills – coaching by adopting a solution-focused approach to help the person move forwards, by developing more effective ways of managing themselves; mentoring as a way of empowering and motivating, by sharing knowledge and teaching; and counselling to help the person deal with distress and other feelings that the effects of making change can provoke. These forms of support are usually accomplished through regular, ongoing meetings.

How you could do this

Part of your support role will be to help the person ensure that actions remain challenging, but are not overwhelming. Often, problems can arise because the person has taken on too much too quickly. They frequently underestimate other demands, which leave them feeling that change is impossible – the odds are stacked against them. They may also lack sufficient feedback. Emotional feedback is particularly important, especially in the early stages, before the person has achieved some success. How they feel can overwhelm the achievement of any goals. An attitude of confidence in their abilities is required while helping the person balance all of these issues.

Good communication is the key to supporting and monitoring someone's progress. The skills needed are the same as those you used before the person made the decision to change. That is, active listening, reflecting meaning, asking mostly open questions, pointing out discrepancies, and summarising. The aim is to help the person gain an insight into their own strengths and limitations and to nurture their ability to resolve difficulties. To do this, and to stop the person taking a resistant stance, continue to explore choices and avoid providing solutions or telling them what to do. In this way, the person remains in control and responsible. Also, avoid generalisations. For a few examples of ineffective and effective feedback, see Figure 14.

Ineffective feedback	More effective feedback
'You need to sort out what you are going to do about ... You won't make any progress until you do.'	'Can you tell me more about the difficulties you are experiencing with ...?'
'You appear to be making good progress.'	'Despite feeling very anxious, you kept going and completed what you set out to do. That shows both determination and courage.'
'What you should do is ...'	'What options are you considering to help with this?'

Figure 14 Ineffective and effective feedback

When giving feedback, it is usually more helpful to:

- ask the person to identify their own strengths from their experience (*'Tell me what you have gained from this experience.'*)

- reinforce these by summarising and adding any further strengths you have identified (*'You have said that you are now able to ... You also said you panicked at one stage and had to use the breathing exercise to regain control. You then went on to ...That shows great courage and that you are gaining control over your feelings in these situations.'*)

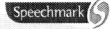

- ask the person to identify any areas of difficulty that need to be addressed ('*Can we talk about how you coped with anything you found uncomfortable or difficult?*' or '*How did you cope with your feelings of anxiety?*')

- discuss these and help the person come up with their own solutions ('*You said that you had some difficulty ... What other tactics could you try using in this situation?*').

There is a tendency for service users to want to rush into and focus immediately on any difficulties they have been experiencing. This sets a negative tone and can negate any positives that are identified later. Identifying positives first sets a progressive tone and helps provide a balanced and solution-focused view of any difficulties encountered. It also avoids the person downplaying their strengths or avoiding difficult issues.

Also, be aware of defensive reactions both from the person you are supporting and from yourself. Here are some examples of defensive reactions from service users:

'It wasn't my fault it didn't work. My wife wouldn't listen.' (Blaming)

'I don't have a problem with that.' (Denial)

'I'm going through a bad time. It happens to everyone.' (Rationalising)

'I don't have to do this!' (Anger)

And here are some defensive reactions that you may be tempted to indulge in:

'I feel it's my duty to tell you ...' (Obligation)

'I'm doing this for your benefit.' (Assuming moral high ground)

'There's no need for you to worry. I will take care of that for you.' (Minimising and taking control)

'I'm sure you're right. I'm making too much of this.' (Colluding)

Make yourself aware when any of these types of defensive statement come into play. They can easily lead to disagreement and to the person becoming argumentative and highly resistant. People feel defensive and/or resistant for a reason. The aim is to find out why and reduce or eliminate the issue. Here are a few responses demonstrating some approaches:

'I sense that you are not completely happy with this. Help me understand what is bothering you.' (Check the cause of any resistance)

'Have you thought about what you are going to do to address this?' (Keep the responsibility and control with the person)

'You seem undecided. You said you felt option three is closest to what you want. What would need to happen to make you feel more comfortable with it?' (Explore possibilities)

'Having looked at what happened, would you accept that, on this occasion, you did lose your temper?' (Help the person to own up to the problem)

'Do you need time to think about this?' (Allow space for the person to absorb and reflect on information)

'Let's return to the strengths you identified earlier and look to see if you can use or build on any of these to help you overcome this difficulty.' (Keep a positive focus)

Comment

The aim is to enable the person to take responsibility for their actions, solve their problems, keep themselves motivated, prevent any resistance to change re-emerging and help them become confident in managing themselves to the point when you are no longer required.

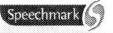

Strategy 28: Sharing knowledge and teaching

Introduction

As part of the process of motivating someone to change and helping them put together an action plan, some skills deficits may be identified that need to be overcome to ensure the plan is successful. How this will be achieved is an essential part of the plan, in order to avoid failure. This need for skills development may be met in different ways – for example, by the person attending an education class or a group in a day centre or other setting. If this is not possible, and you have the knowledge and skills to do so, you may need to put together a teaching programme to meet the need.

How you could do this

You will need, first, to assess which skills or aspects of skills need reinforcing. For example, if the person has difficulty forming relationships, this may be because they have poor knowledge of the basic rules of social interaction. In this instance, you will need to explore which aspects they find problematic. This could be being able to chat to people, or they may have difficulty forming deeper relationships or be unaware of the rules that govern particular situations; they may be shy or lack confidence, and so on. It would also be worth learning what the person wants from their relationships. What skills will they need to obtain this?

Once you are aware of what skills need to be developed, you can then decide what training is required and whether it is appropriate for you to carry that out or whether it can be addressed in another way – perhaps by reading or attending a class.

If you decide you will carry out the training, you will need to put together a programme to do this. If it is a social skills matter, this might include demonstrating and role-playing situations as a means of teaching verbal and non-verbal communication. To address shyness issues, you might

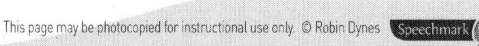

teach the person some relaxation methods and work with them on systematic desensitisation. Do not act alone when drawing up these programmes: consult with your supervisor, colleagues and other professionals. Most will be only too pleased to share their knowledge, experience and ideas. You may also need their assistance to help with role play, and so on.

Often, the skills required to make a significant difference can be taught in one or two sessions.

Comment

In some types of setting, such as residential or day centres, finding time to engage with people in this way can be difficult because of the pressure of the number of tasks to be completed each day. However, it is worth it. After all, if a person is expected to change some unacceptable or maladaptive behaviour, they need to be taught the skills to be able to do that. In the long term, the time saved by enabling the person to cope and to manage their situation will more than compensate. You will also gain satisfaction and pleasure from their accomplishment.

Strategy 29: Time management

Introduction

One of the self-managing skills people often need some help with is managing their time. This may come to light if they make statements such as: *'Oh, I didn't have time to do anything'* or *'I'm too busy to be able to do this.'* There may be various reasons for these statements. If you have explored the issue with them, and discovered they are having difficulty managing time, then this will need to be addressed.

How you could do this

You may encounter some barriers and resistance to managing time. These can include:

'I will be committed to doing things I don't like all day.'

'I won't have time to relax or get involved in social activities.'

'I feel guilty if I'm not doing something.'

'I won't be able to do it. I don't have time.'

'I like to be involved in everything. I hate missing out.'

'I constantly feel stressed and tired out. I always seem to be struggling to keep up.'

Of course, the effective management of time addresses all of these types of issue. Point this out and encourage the person by saying something like:

'Let's explore this and then you decide if you think it would help.'

If they agree, you can then invite them to go through their typical week and write down all the tasks they do each day, from when they get up until they go to bed. (Recording how they spend time can be given as an exercise for a follow-up meeting.) Include as much as possible: time taken in the bathroom, having breakfast, cleaning the house, listening to music, phoning friends, shopping, going for a walk, watching television, cooking meals, doing the washing, having a rest or relaxing, working, indulging in a hobby, doing nothing, and so on. Once completed, this will give a good indication of how the person spends their time and whether there are any gaps that could be filled by completing tasks on their plan for change.

Sometimes activities can be rearranged to make better use of time and to make space in daily routines for other activities or personal time. When doing this, the person may discover that they are continuing to do things which are no longer necessary and of no importance. They can then decide whether they want to stop doing those things. If a day is absolutely packed with activities, the person will need to decide what is the most important for them to do, or whether some of those activities could be carried out on a different day. When assisting people to plan their week, encourage them to allow gaps for the unexpected, to have time for themselves, and to create a fair balance between doing those things that are necessary and the things they enjoy.

Comment

Completing the process above often produces surprises for individuals about how they use time. Help the person to identify what is important to them and what is not. You may need to highlight discrepancies by using reflections and summarising points which are incongruent and not in line with their beliefs and goals. Be careful to ensure that no judgemental or impatient tone creeps into your voice and that the emphasis is always on the person being in control of any decisions.

Strategy 30: Understanding self-talk

Introduction

Becoming aware of the conversations that we have with ourselves is essential when making changes or being confronted with difficulties and problems. What we believe and tell ourselves has a powerful effect on whether or not we keep going and what we achieve. These thoughts are referred to as 'self-talk'. This self-talk is often not realistic or constructive and can be a barrier that feeds resistance and diminishes confidence and self-esteem. It is important to remember, when raising awareness of self-talk and how it can be used to help rather than hinder progress, that the person will have been talking to themselves in a particular way for a long time. Changing an old habit can take time.

How you could do this

The first step is to help the person recognise the chatter that is going on in their head and differentiate between what is helpful and what is not. Unhelpful thoughts are those which are negative and which discourage and hinder progress. Helpful thoughts are realistic, non-judgemental, supportive and encouraging and reinforce the person's ability to achieve their goals. They are, in fact, the qualities you, or a coach, would use when listening to the person and supporting them to achieve their goals. Figure 15 lists some examples of both unhelpful and helpful chatter.

Unhelpful chatter	Helpful chatter
'I can't do this.'	'This is difficult but if I take it a step at a time, I will get there.'
'I've made an effort but it isn't working. I might as well give up.'	'This method is not working for me. Perhaps I could try ...'
'I can't do anything right.'	'It's OK to make mistakes. I don't need to be perfect.'
'My friends will ridicule me.'	'If they don't wish me well, they are not really good friends. Anyway, I can cope with a bit of good-natured mickey-taking.'
'It will be too embarrassing. I won't do it.'	'I will feel uncomfortable at first but that will fade. People will appreciate my honesty.'
'Who do you think you are? You're not important.'	'I have the same rights as everyone else. What I want is just as important.'
'I'm not ready to do this yet.'	'Stop using delaying tactics. You're afraid of failing. Make a start now and learn from the experience.'
'I'll do it sometime during the week.'	'Stop putting this off. Be specific. I'll do this at 2pm today.'
'This is hopeless. I've done nothing this week.'	'This week I have thought about and decided what I will do about ... I made an appointment to see ... I talked to my Mum. She will support me by ...'

Figure 15 Unhelpful and helpful chatter

You can help the person isolate the unhelpful chatter by inviting them to write down unhelpful thoughts that they regularly experience. If they have difficulty with this, ask them to record the thoughts during the day or week as they occur. They can do this in a diary or a notebook. Once you have a list of unhelpful thoughts and thinking habits, ask them to come up with alternative, more helpful statements they could use instead. Although you may need to make suggestions, this strategy is most effective when the person comes up with their own alternative and uses their own words. You can encourage this by using comments such as:

'If you were advising a friend, what would you say to them?'

'What do you think would be most helpful to be saying to yourself?'

'If you felt more confident, what might you be saying to yourself?'

Sometimes individuals will say *'Oh, but I am hopeless.'* If they do, then you will need to help them examine the evidence to justify these thoughts. For example, the person may say, *'I can't get anything right.'* You can then go through everything they have done that day and find that, out of all those things, they got one thing wrong – certainly not justification for labelling themselves with such a negative thought and for thinking about themselves in that way.

The helpful statements, when compiled, should be rehearsed vocally by the person and written in their notebook or on cards. When the unhelpful thoughts occur, they can then take out their notebook if necessary and substitute the more helpful thoughts. With constant repetition, the process of stopping unhelpful thoughts and substituting helpful ones will become habitual.

Comment

Teaching the person to listen to and make use of self-talk in this way enables them to begin coaching themselves, believe in their ability to achieve, look at their options creatively and keep focused, and acknowledges their achievements. It has a really positive effect on their outlook and self-esteem.

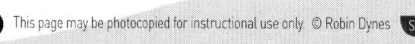

Strategy 31: Dealing with emotions

Introduction

Dealing with people inevitably means dealing with emotions. It is the part of making changes with which the person is most likely to struggle. This makes it important to be able to recognise feelings and detect their more subtle influences as well as those which are very obvious. Our own sensitivity can sometimes be blunted when we are under pressure or preoccupied with our own thoughts. We might also feel satisfaction that the person has a good plan and is well supported, but that they just need to get on with putting the plan into action and ignore any emotional reaction. These feelings we are experiencing influence our responses, which might be those of impatience or of ignoring signs that the person is struggling to deal with the emotional effects of taking action. Therefore, great care needs to be taken over how we deal with our own emotions as well as those of the person with whom we are working.

How you could do this

Frequently, the person will express their feelings openly and it would be extremely difficult not to recognise them. When this happens, it can be tempting to listen briefly, acknowledge those feelings by saying something like: *'I know how you feel'*, and attempt to move on. This can lead to a strong reaction because the person may construe from this that their feelings have been invalidated and ignored. Even if they do not react strongly, such a response will tend to alienate and distance the person. It is better to respond with a statement which recognises and validates the emotions expressed, such as:

'I can see that this is upsetting ...'

'I realise that you must be feeling angry.'

'I recognise how frustrating this must be for you.'

'I see you are really pleased with ...'

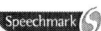

This avoids giving the impression that you know what is going on inside the person's head and alienating them, and allows you to follow through, using active listening skills.

Lambert (1996) provides a mnemonic as a reminder of what to do when there are signs of heightened emotions, which is illustrated in Figure 16. (Lambert's mnemonic is in the first column; the comments in the second column are by the author of this book.)

S – Stop talking	If the person shows signs of becoming agitated, angry or tearful, stop talking and start listening. This will calm things down and show that you are taking the person's feelings seriously.
A – Active listening	Show through body language and short comments ('*Go on ...*', '*Tell me more ...*') that you are listening actively. Make it clear that you are focusing on the person, taking the matter seriously and trying to understand.
R – Reflect content or feeling	This entails reflecting back your understanding of the situation. This may involve summarising the main issues so the person can verify you have understood correctly ('*Am I correct in thinking that ...?*', '*Let me see if I have got this right ...*').
A – Act with empathy	Recognise and acknowledge how the person is feeling ('*I can see you are very angry*'). This does not mean that you feel the same way – angry, sad, joyful, frustrated or irritated. Feeling the same way may inadvertently further inflame how the person feels.
H – Handle objections	Having calmed the situation down, the person is now more likely to listen to reason and be able to move towards exploring a solution to their problem. Do not give in to temptation to provide ready-made actions. To avoid objections and resistance, the solution is best generated by the person themselves: ('*Have you thought about what you would like to do about this?*' or '*What has helped in the past when you have felt like this?*'

Figure 16 Guide to Handling Emotions (Source: Lambert, 1996)

When dealing with emotion, it is helpful to be aware of the distinction between sympathy and empathy. Being sympathetic means you share the same feelings as the other person in their particular circumstances. Being empathetic means that you recognise the other person's feelings, such as sadness, guilt or irritation, without feeling them yourself – and responding in an appropriate way. However, it is only human to feel something of what the other person is experiencing.

If you were to take on all the feelings of the people you deal with in care situations, you would quickly become swamped and overwhelmed by it all. The aim is to be sensitive to people's emotions: to be empathetic but to avoid allowing sympathy to hamper your effectiveness.

Staying aware and responding to other people's feelings is complex and demanding. Different emotions require different approaches. During the process of change, individuals can experience a wide range and intensity of feelings, including those shown in Figure 17 (overleaf).

 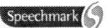

Loss	This may be the loss of a familiar way of life, or friends, or security.
Anger	This is anger or frustration the person directs at themselves or other people because something has not worked out as expected.
Joy	Expression of joy at successful achievements can result in overenthusiasm, unrealistic expectations and the person overestimating their abilities. The person may need to be helped to adopt a more realistic perspective to avoid disappointment.
Anxiety	This may be a sense of discomfort, unease or fear about doing something new or taking responsibility, or about what achieving their goals will mean.
Guilt	The person may feel that by making changes they are deserting or letting someone down. Guilt can be an irrational response to making a painful break with some past habits, behaviour, way of life or people.

Figure 17 Feelings experienced during change

Often, you will detect subtle indications of emotions through body language. They may be shown through a shrug, the tone of voice, the way the person is sitting, agitated body movements such as foot shaking, finger tapping, grimacing, and so on. These indications can be approached by statements such as:

'I sense you feel unhappy about ...'

'Has something happened that has upset you?'

'You look disappointed with what you have achieved.'

'I can see you are really pleased with your success. Tell me about it.'

Comment

It is difficult to predict what emotions will arise when dealing with a range of people. Do remember that acknowledging and validating emotions of joy and pleasure at success are just as important as acknowledging sadness, frustration, and so on. Focus on listening to fears and anxieties and on providing choices rather than solutions. Doing this helps build confidence and self-esteem.

As well as the person you are working with experiencing hope, joy, irritation, anxiety, doubts, feelings of inadequacy, and so on, you will also be experiencing those emotions. For this reason, and to help you deal with these emotions so they do not interfere with what you are doing, it is important that you have a good supervision and support system in place which you can use to obtain advice and guidance to help you sort out your own thinking and feelings. Also, be aware of the limitations of your skills and refer people on to appropriately qualified professionals as necessary.

Strategy 32: Monitoring progress

Introduction

Events rarely go exactly as planned. The unexpected happens, difficulties arise and choices for action turn out not to be as effective as first thought. Other things go better than expected and individuals are surprised by their success. There are lots of ups and downs when working towards a goal. Part of your supporting role will be to help the person learn how to monitor their own progress, deal with the issues that arise and resolve any problems.

How you could do this

While doing this, you may use different communication styles. In their book *Motivational Interviewing in Health Care*, Rollnick *et al* (2008) refer to these as 'directing', 'following' and 'guiding' (see Figure 18 – the comments in the right-hand column are by the author of this book).

During different times and in different situations you might use any of these styles. Rather than adopt one, you are likely to move fluidly from one to another, as appropriate.

A good approach when monitoring progress is to use Kolb's (1984) learning cycle as a pattern to help the person learn from their experiences (see Figure 19).

Directing	When using this style you are in charge. You might adopt this style when there is an emergency situation or when you are providing expertise, information or teaching. The person is dependent on you to make decisions and for advice and action.
Following	When using this style you follow the person's lead. You listen and try to understand the situation, focusing on how the person sees the problem and avoiding giving advice. The person is in charge and you move at their pace. This style is particularly useful when responding to highly emotional reactions.
Guiding	You would adopt this style when working in collaboration with a service user. You might point out options for dealing with difficulties, solving problems and highlighting risks, and explain the benefits of choices, and so on. You assist the person in choosing the best options, but they remain in charge and responsible for their decisions.

Figure 18 Directing, following and guiding

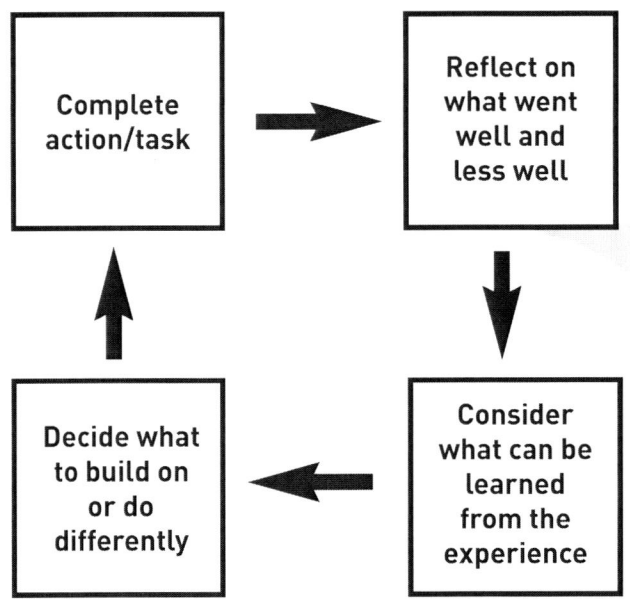

Figure19 Kolb's learning cycle (Source: adapted from Kolb, 1984)

Following this process enables the person to learn from their experience, adopt an approach and attitude that is positive, and avoid feeling a failure because actions have not worked out or been as successful as they had hoped. It also gives the opportunity to acknowledge and plan to celebrate what has gone well. It is easy for the person to bring up issues that bother them. You can identify and explore any discrepancies that appear. While working through the steps, you can maintain a motivational approach that is encouraging, and the person will have learned a process that will serve them well in all walks of life.

Keeping a journal

One way to aid someone to incorporate this process into their lifestyle, and to use it in monitoring sessions, is to encourage them to keep a journal. Using their goals, and their plans for achieving them, as a guide, each day they record what happens as they carry out their planned actions. Entries may include:

- any traps fallen into, such as negative self-talk

- what has gone well and how they feel when it does

- what has not gone so well, and their reactions and feelings

- feedback from other people

- any incidents or problems and how they managed them

- anything they did to keep going and to stay motivated and positive.

Completing this journal need only take a few minutes towards the end of each day. Then, at the end of the week or at a planned monitoring session, the person reads through their notes and reflects on the week, what they did, what has been achieved, what they have learned, and what further actions and adjustments need to be made to build on their experience. If they are doing this on their own, they will need to remember to acknowledge, congratulate and reward themselves for what they have achieved. This includes having the courage and putting the effort into trying out an action, even if on previous occasions it has not been completely successful.

Emphasise to the person that completing their journal need only take a few minutes each day and around 15 minutes or so at the end of the week. Once the habit is formed, the process becomes automatic and they will find themselves doing it in their head instinctively.

Comment

Enabling the person to monitor their own progress, take control of their own learning and resolve difficulties gives them a skill for life, not just one that will help them deal with their current difficulties. It also equips the person to eventually feel confident that they can manage without your support.

Strategy 33: Providing feedback

Introduction

Providing feedback on progress is another essential task within the supporting role. Many people perceive the concept of feedback as being critical and judgemental. This can create considerable discomfort and anxiety. They might have experienced feedback in the past that was critical or negative or given as an evaluation of abilities, and they may, consequently, have good reason to fear and shun feedback now.

Absence of feedback deprives the person of the opportunity to learn from experience and develop and achieve their goals. If given badly, it can kill both enthusiasm and motivation, resulting in the person becoming highly resistant. The aim is to provide both positive and negative feedback in a spirit of unconditional positive regard and in a way that is clearly designed to help improve the learner's performance (Dobbie & Tysinger, 2005).

How you could do this

Johari's Window (Luft, 1969) is a good model for receiving and giving feedback. It was developed by two psychologists – Joseph Luft and Harry Ingram – hence the name Johari, which is pronounced 'Joeharry'. The tool looks like a window (see Figure 20). It also uses the metaphor of a window, as it is a way of looking at ourselves and others. It divides knowledge about ourselves into four panes or areas.

	Things you know about yourself	Things you do not know about yourself
Things others know about you	**PUBLIC AREA** Sometimes called the 'open' area. It consists of things you know about yourself and know that other people know about you. *(The colour of your eyes, that you have three children, etc.)*	**BLIND AREA** This is what is known to other people but not obvious or admitted to yourself. *(Perhaps that you are seen as kind or stubborn.)*
Things others do not know about you	**HIDDEN AREA** These are the things you know about yourself but choose not to tell other people. *(You dislike a gift you have been given, you cheated in an exam or gave a large donation to a local charity, you fear losing control.)*	**UNKNOWN AREA** This covers what you do not know or do not recognise about yourself and is also not known by others. *(This might be abilities and potential that you have not yet discovered about yourself, such as that you have a natural talent for organising or decorating.)*

Figure 20 Johari's Window (Source: adapted from Luft, 1969)

In reality, the areas are not quite so static or neat. Information can move from one pane to another as mutual trust is built and more information is shared. Also, often what we think is hidden from others may be obvious to them through our body language and how we act, without us being aware of it. Conversely, things we think should be obvious to others are, in fact, hidden. In addition, people make assumptions or judgements about each other based on their own experience and what they think they know,

 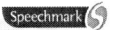

which may or may not be true. Guarding against doing this is essential when supporting someone and giving feedback. Keep in mind too that the other person will probably be making assumptions about you.

This is why it is so important to check when communicating both your understanding of what has been said and that the other person has correctly understood your meaning.

When you first begin working with an individual, you will start by drawing out as much information as possible. This expands the 'public area' known to you and what you have observed during this process (the 'blind area'). The idea is then to expand the person's knowledge further, by giving feedback about what they are not aware of (the 'blind area'), thus expanding their 'public' window of knowledge. By working together and asking questions which encourage self-exploration, you can also help the person shrink the 'hidden' and 'unknown' areas. Thus, as their window of knowledge about themselves is increased, they are motivated and empowered to make changes.

This would seem to indicate that communication is likely to be most effective when everyone is operating within the 'public area'. If so, should our aim then be to always be like an 'open book', telling everyone everything about ourselves? The answer is 'No'. Context dictates what is appropriate and what is not. If in a close and intimate relationship, the 'public area' between the two people involved will be large. If chatting to someone who is an acquaintance through sharing a hobby, it may only be appropriate to share general information and knowledge about the hobby. When working with an individual and giving feedback on their progress, you would operate within the context of the person achieving their goal.

Principles for giving feedback

1 **Reflecting on what went well and less well**. Keeping Kolb's learning cycle in mind (see Strategy 32: 'Monitoring progress'), ask about and listen to the experience of the person and how they view their progress. If you have previously asked the person the question, *'How will you know when you have succeeded?'* before they carried out a particular action or step, they will have something to measure their success against. Encourage them to be specific and to express how they felt when taking any actions. If they make general comments, such as *'It went well'* or *'It was awful'*, enquire how it went well or badly: *'What did you do? Describe how you were feeling. What thoughts were going through your head? Tell me what strengths this shows.'* Using your active listening skills, reflect and summarise the main points, focusing on and affirming the positives.

2 **Considering what can be learned from the experience**. Discuss the difference between what the person set out to achieve and what actually happened. Were their expectations realistic? What have they learned from the experience? From the discussion and your observations, are there things within the 'blind', 'hidden' or 'unknown' areas which can be used to expand their knowledge about themselves? (These could be courage, fear of success, a belief that is based on misinformation, an unacknowledged skill which has been demonstrated, potential exposed, and so on.)

This is a joint discussion in which both parties actively contribute. Again, use open questions, reflection and summarising skills related to the learning cycle to draw out and support self-motivating statements and belief in change. Ask the person to summarise what has been learned: *'What do you feel you have learned from this experience?'* Discuss and add anything which they have not acknowledged and highlight any inconsistencies.

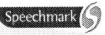

3 **Deciding what to build on or do differently**. Help the person to think of ways in which they can build on their experience and to practise needed skills. If one approach they have tried does not work for them, guide them towards using a different method: *'What else might help you ...?'*, *'Can you think of another way that might work better for you?'*, or *'Another service user tried ... Could that work for you?'* This part of the feedback session clarifies and reinforces what has been achieved and enables the person to plan the actions that are now needed in order to build on this achievement and move forwards.

This learning cycle is a process which is repeated time and time again as the person progresses towards achieving their goals. Take care to use non-judgemental language which is specific and solution-focused and easily understood by the person. Concentrate on observed behaviours rather than on personal characteristics. Instead of saying: *'You acted in an aggressive manner during the role play'*, say something like: *'When we did the role play, your voice was loud and had an aggressive and threatening tone. Your facial expression and the way you pointed at my chest also indicated aggression rather than assertiveness. What could you do differently to avoid coming across as aggressive?'*

Comment

Having obtained the service user's permission, in some instances – such as role play – you may be able to use sound recordings or videos to further enhance feedback and the person's knowledge about themselves. Do be aware, however, that, for some people, seeing and hearing themselves can be a very uncomfortable experience. Making sure they know the recording will be destroyed and letting them witness this happening can help to allay fears.

Strategy 34: Using a support network

Introduction

Having a good support system in place can have a really positive effect on helping a person achieve and it can be a crucial factor in helping them succeed. Some people will have lots of friends, but that does not mean that all of those people will support or have an interest in someone achieving their goals. In fact, some so-called friends may exercise a negative influence and derive benefit if the person fails. For these reasons, depending on what is to be achieved, it may be worth helping the person examine their support system and ensuring that appropriate support is incorporated into any plan.

How you could do this

The leading question here is: *'Who do you think would support you in achieving this goal?'* It is also worth checking the person's understanding of how other people can help them: *'What do you think would be the benefits of telling chosen people what you are doing, and how might it help you?'* Ensure that the benefits discussed include having someone to:

- provide encouragement
- talk to when needed
- help the person keep to commitments
- have fun with
- help when they feel stressed
- suggest solutions to problems encountered.

When the person agrees that they will benefit from using a support network, invite them to write a list of those who could support them and how they might do this. For an example, see Figure 21 (overleaf).

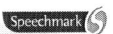

Who might help	How they could help	What I can do in return
Mum	Remind me about and make sure I attend appointments	Trim the hedges and cut the grass regularly
Peter (best friend)	Cheer me up when I am feeling low and help me celebrate successes	Support him when he is playing football
Jane (girlfriend)	Talk things through with me and make helpful suggestions	Go with her and push the wheelchair when she takes her disabled mother shopping
Brother	Keep me focused on what I am doing and encourage me	Listen to the problems he has at work and make helpful suggestions
Support worker	Help me monitor my progress and resolve difficulties	Turn up for appointments on time

Figure 21 Planning a support network

When the list is being compiled, keep the person focused on key issues that are relevant to success. Remind them that friendship and obtaining support is a two-way process: they should also consider what they can do for the person supporting them. They may not always be able to do anything in return immediately, but they should keep it in mind for the future. Once the list is complete, it is helpful for the person to consider what other help would be useful and how they might obtain it. This will depend on each individual situation and might include people such as their:

• tutor

• landlord

- manager

- doctor

- religious leader

- nurse

- probation officer.

Once it has been established who might help, they will then need to plan how they will approach the person or people and clarify how they would like to be supported by them. Remind individuals that it is not a trading situation – that is, it is not a matter of *'If you do this for me, I will do this for you.'* It needs to be approached with more subtlety: *'Is there anything I can do to help you?'* or *'I thought it might help you if I ...'* Most people will be pleased to give support and may be offended if the person making the request adopts a trading attitude.

Also, remind individuals that the person approached has the right to say *'No'*. If they do, this should be respected in a gracious manner: *'Thank you for listening to me and considering my request.'* They will then need to decide on someone else for that particular role.

Comment

During the process of establishing appropriate support, you will still need to use your active listening skills and you may need to highlight some inconsistencies: *'You said John drinks a lot and gets funny when you don't. This results in you getting drunk. How does that fit with using him to support you in controlling your drinking?'*

 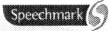

SECTION 5

Ensuring momentum is maintained (Maintenance)

Once change has been achieved and old habits have been broken, the person needs to acknowledge that they are still vulnerable. They need to review their initial goals and set new ones, make adjustments, avoid overconfidence, check their thinking, and guard against slipping back.

Strategy 35: Reviewing and resetting goals

Introduction

Once actions have been taken and initial goals have been achieved, there is a danger that the person making the changes relaxes and feels that is the end of the matter. For example, a person may keep to a diet to reduce weight. When they reach their target, they relax and gradually start putting weight back on again. The same might apply to an undesirable behaviour. To avoid this happening, the person needs to review their initial goals and set new ones.

How you could do this

Life presents us with continuous change – ageing, unforeseen circumstances, accidents, children leaving home, caring for elderly parents, and so on. As we progress through it, we have to adapt. As we achieve one goal and situations change, we need to review what has happened and set new goals to suit the new circumstances. To continue with the example above, a person might have achieved their target weight loss. Do they continue with their present diet and lose more weight or should they set themselves a new target to maintain their target weight? To maintain their desired weight, they will need a new goal and a plan to achieve that.

First, they need to decide what their new goal will be, bearing in mind it needs to be **SMART**: that is, **S**pecific, **M**easurable, **A**ppealing, **R**ealistic and **T**ime limited (see Strategy 23: 'Negotiating goals'). Then, to help them plan how this will be achieved, they will need to review what strategies worked well previously, which less well, and what they have learned from their experience (see Kolb's learning cycle in Strategy 32: 'Monitoring progress'). A simple form such as that shown in Figure 22 can be used to do this. This information can then be used to plan the steps needed to achieve the new goals (see Strategy 24:'Planning the change' for suggestions on how to do this).

STRATEGY REVIEW FORM		
What worked well?	What worked less well?	What I have learned from experience?

Figure 22 Example of a strategy review form

Comment

When it comes to setting new goals, you may encounter some resistance. The person may feel that there is no need. You will detect this in their body language, their attitude, what they say and how they say it. The person may be feeling overconfident or that setting new goals is not necessary. The danger here is that they will gradually drift back into old habits. You will need to apply the same tactics as you did initially: using listening skills, open-ended questions, paraphrasing, reflecting meaning, and highlighting discrepancies in thinking, while avoiding arguing.
It remains essential that the person still feels totally in control of what they do.

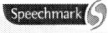

Strategy 36: Ensuring change is permanent

Introduction

Having achieved the original goals and set new targets, it is very easy, and natural, for the person to feel satisfied and let down their guard. Early warning signs may not be as strong as losing their temper, stopping exercising or eating the wrong foods but, rather, a gradual lessening of commitment. Friends who have supported the service user may feel that it is no longer necessary or the person may slowly begin to expose themselves to situations and environments that tempt them back into old behaviours. These dangers need to be guarded against.

How you could do this

Make the person aware of the dangers. They may vaguely have them in the back of their mind but ignore them, thinking: *'Oh, I've got this under control now. Life's too short. I can enjoy myself this once.'* Ask them: *'What do you think the dangers are going to be for you in ensuring you maintain your new way of life?'* You can help them with this by getting them to review the difficulties they encountered when making the changes and how they overcame them. Encourage them to make a list. Use a format similar to that shown in Figure 23.

MAINTAINING CHANGE	
Dangers to maintaining change	**How I can cope with these dangers**

Figure 23 Example of a maintaining change form

They can then look at this form from time to time, to remind themselves of the dangers and how they coped with the difficulty in the past.

Another useful method of reinforcing their commitment to maintaining change is to revisit what were the negative aspects of their old behaviour and way of life. Why did they want to make the change? What are the benefits of having changed? Again, this may be done using a simple list (see Figure 24) which the person can keep and look at to remind themselves and maintain commitment.

MAINTAINING COMMITMENT TO CHANGE	
Negative aspects of my old behaviour/way of life	Benefits of having changed

Figure 24 Example of a maintaining commitment to change form

Accepting responsibility

Encourage the person to accept responsibility for their own success and to celebrate it from time to time. Often, people attribute their success to others – these might be a support worker, friends, their partner, and so on. When they do this, they undermine their confidence and ability and their commitment to success. They should acknowledge the support and help given by others, but they need to accept responsibility for their own success. An inclination on their part to minimise their achievement may be picked up in what they say and how they say it: *'My success is down to my partner.'* These sorts of statements and other indications of attributing

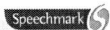

their success to others need to be challenged. The other person may have contributed, but the success needs to be owned by the person who has made the change. Do this by getting them to summarise the actions they took, then ask: *'Having done all this, who do you think is responsible for your success?'* Reinforce the answer by stating that you also believe they are responsible and should be proud of their achievement.

Celebrating achievements

One way to show acceptance of responsibility for personal success and to reinforce commitment is, at set intervals, to celebrate success. The person can set times to do this – on their birthday, at New Year, at six-monthly intervals, on the anniversary of when they made the change, for example. On these occasions they can review how it is going and any dangers or new difficulties encountered and resolved, make adjustments to their goals, and remind themselves about the negative aspects of their old behaviour and the benefits they now enjoy. They can celebrate in a way appropriate to maintaining their goals, either privately or with someone else.

Maintaining a support network

After initial goals have been achieved, it is likely that some members of the person's support system will consider themselves no longer necessary. The person will need to renew their agreement with some of those who have given support in the past. They may need to adjust these agreements to the new situation. Professionals such as doctors, nurses or social workers may decide their support is no longer needed. However, having an agreement with a partner, relative or friend to continue their support, or to remind the person when they are in danger of relapse, will help reinforce commitment and maintain the new behaviour.

Check self-talk

How the person uses self-talk (see Strategy 30: 'Understanding self-talk') can begin to lapse. The problems of the past can begin to fade and seem less threatening. The person may also start to minimise the effects their behaviour was having on their lives and the lives of others. Self-talk may begin to resemble: *'Well, it wasn't that bad'*, *'My behaviour didn't really harm anyone'*, *'My lack of assertiveness wasn't really much of a problem'* or *'My anger wasn't really out of control.'*

These types of thoughts weaken commitment and can lead to relapse. To avoid this happening, individuals need to periodically check their self-talk. They might also ask supporters to remind them just how much their behaviour was affecting their life and the lives of others. They could also look back to the negative aspects of their previous behaviour or way of life. This will help them avoid distorting or rationalising the past.

They can realign their thinking and come up with more useful thoughts which own and acknowledge past behaviour and are more realistic and helpful. For example: *'Yes, I did have an anger problem. Not addressing it would have ended in my marriage breaking up. Using the strategies I learned ensures the future security of my marriage.'* These more helpful thoughts can be written down, learned and looked at again and again, as necessary.

Comment

It is only human for people to make mistakes, have slip-ups and be tempted with a longing for some aspect of their past behaviour. This may be for a way of life or to be involved in a situation that opens up temptations, to eat an unhealthy diet or revert to unacceptable behaviour. The solution is to learn from slip-ups and guard against them becoming a serious relapse.

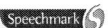

Strategy 37: Coping with anxiety and stress

Introduction

Life and events do not always go as we expect. Unexpected things sometimes occur which cannot be foreseen. We have to deal with ups and downs – sometimes feeling on top of the world, sometimes disappointed, frustrated, anxious, stressed and even that everything is too much. These are normal feelings. The service user may need to learn some strategies to help them cope with these feelings.

How you could do this

First, ask the person: *'What has helped you with this in the past?'* If this does not produce satisfactory solutions, there are a number of strategies you could suggest including the following:

- Talk things through with a friend or someone you trust. (This may be someone who supports them and to whom they have given this role. See Strategy 34: 'Using a support network'.)

- Learn and practise some relaxation techniques to use when you are feeling stressed. (You may need to teach the person some methods – guided breathing, progressive muscle relaxation or meditation – which suit. Some are available online via computers, smartphones and other electronic devices. The person may also find that listening to a particular type of music helps them relax. Classes may be available or relaxation recordings could be obtained.)

- Deal with problems as soon as possible. Take control and avoid them building up.

- Divert your attention. Do something you enjoy – paint, write, read or do some gardening. Take up a hobby. For example, learn how to play a musical instrument or compile your family history.

- Do some sort of exercise – go for a walk or a swim, play table tennis or take up a sport. Make it something you enjoy. (Elicit this by asking what the person has done in the past that they enjoyed. It may also be helpful for them to do an activity with one of their supporters or a friend.)

- Examine your use of time (see Strategy 29: 'Time management'). Are you trying to do too much or are there periods in which you do nothing? Either of these can cause stress. Do you have a balance between doing what is essential and what you enjoy doing? Have you allowed time for yourself?

- Be aware of your self-talk (also see Strategy 30: 'Understanding self-talk). Monitor the voice in your head that is adding out-of-proportion fears, worries, self-criticism or guilt to what you are already feeling. Substitute more encouraging thoughts and coach yourself through the moment as if you were your own best friend. (The person may have given a supporter the role of helping them challenge and substitute more helpful thoughts. See Strategy 34: 'Using a support network'.)

- Live in the here-and-now rather than letting automatic self-talk take control. Take things one step at a time. Stop criticising or questioning your past actions or decisions or worrying about the future when, in fact, everything is OK in the present. Accept the past – you cannot change it – and remind yourself that it is pointless to worry about out-of-proportion fears concerning events in the future that may never happen.

- Take actions which are guided by your beliefs, values and goals (see Strategy 5:'Establishing values and beliefs'). This means having the courage 'to do what it takes', although that may not always feel comfortable. Talk through a problem with a supporter. Say 'No' when you need to do so, to avoid putting yourself in a situation that could cause you problems. Ask for help when you need it.

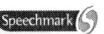

- Accept yourself as you are, with all your perceived flaws and shortcomings, as being just as valuable as anyone else. You are worth while just because you are human and, like everyone else, you are just trying to live as best you can and achieve what you want from life (Edelman, 2002). Focus on what you need to do now and not on some perfectionist ideas about the future (Reynolds, 2002).

Comment

The strategies listed above need to be presented to the person in a way that makes them acceptable and to avoid them being resisted. For example: *'Have you thought of examining how you use time? Would you like to do that now to see if it shows up anything that might help?'* or *'Some people find that doing some exercise helps in these types of circumstance. You said you have enjoyed swimming in the past. What do you think about going for a swim when you feel ... to see if it helps?'* It makes it easier if you think through each suggestion and then practise how you might present it.

Strategy 38: Techniques for staying motivated

Introduction

Once you have encouraged someone to make some changes, set goals and take some action, you may need to equip them with some suggestions to help them stay motivated. Some people will find that once they have succeeded with the first few steps, enough momentum will have been created to spur them on. However, when difficulties, obstructions, tedium and life intervene with diversions, they may stumble and begin to lose enthusiasm. Ensure that the person has some strategies built into their action plan that will help when this happens.

How you could do this

As with Strategy 37: 'Coping with anxiety and stress', asking the question *'What has helped you stay motivated in the past?'* is a good place to start. If the person has difficulty identifying strategies that worked for them, here are a few you could suggest.

- Reward themselves in some way for each step achieved: rewards should be included in their action plan. It gives them something to look forward to, acknowledges their success, and reinforces forward movement.

- Begin by setting targets which are fairly easy to achieve. Also, if a planned step seems overwhelming, encourage them to break it down into smaller units. This will seem less daunting and once the first actions have been taken, the person will then feel more motivated to continue.

- Explore how they feel about moving out of their comfort zone and taking risks. When we try something new, it does not always feel comfortable at first, nor does it always work as anticipated. Even if a

 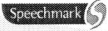

step has not worked well, the person can tell themselves:
'This didn't work as well as I thought. However, I have shown courage and determination and I learned I need to try a different approach. That makes the effort well worth while.'

- Have quiet moments when they imagine what success will feel like. How will they feel when they have achieved their goals? What will life be like? What will they be doing? They can visualise it, using all their senses.

- Create a symbol for themselves to remind them of their strengths when their resolve begins to weaken. This might be a solid oak tree when their determination begins to falter, or a lion, with its courage and tenacity.

- Use their sense of humour: laugh at themselves and their idiosyncrasy. Being able to see the comical side of something can enable the person to put it into perspective and prevent it from diminishing motivation.

- Praise themselves regularly: *'I was dreading that but I managed to do it anyway. Well done!'* or *'I made a good job of that.'* They might keep a diary in which they record each achievement and praise themselves for it. They can then use this as a reminder of their successes.

- Take a few minutes to refocus and coach themselves if they do not feel like doing something or they are drifting from their goals. They can remind themselves about their goals and imagine what they would say if they were coaching their best friend: *'You need to put your health first. Spend the next 15 minutes exercising as planned. You can record the television programme and watch it later.'*

- Think of their goal as a long journey and their current slump as just a dip in the road. People do not give up because of a dip. There will be some hills to climb, some valleys to cross and some long, boring flat bits, just as there will be exhilarating, exciting and fun bits. Encourage them to stick with it, ride out the ups and downs and they will get there.

- Keep the benefits constantly in mind: instead of thinking about the difficulties and how hard something is going to be, they should think about the benefits. For example, rather than thinking how hard it will be to do exercises regularly and keep to a diet, refocus on how good they will feel when they have lost weight. Substituting the unhelpful thoughts for helpful ones will create energy and enthusiasm.

- Make friends with people who are positive and supportive. Being with people who are negative and critical will eat away at their resolve. Being with people who are supportive will encourage and help sustain a positive attitude.

- Treat mistakes and diversions from their chosen path as opportunities to learn: *'I now know that doing ... doesn't work for me. Next time I will try ... '* and *'How can I improve on this?'*

Comment

Everyone is different. What motivates one person may not work with another. What helps in one situation may not help in another. Most people will use different tactics at different times.

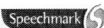

Strategy 39: Understanding what people say

Introduction

How people use words to explain their experiences has a powerful effect on the meaning they convey, whether or not they are understood and how they cope with and overcome difficulties encountered. It can also have a profound effect on how enthusiastic and motivated they feel from day to day. Look out for weaknesses in thinking and communication and help the person to be more specific about what they mean, by using language in a way that is more supportive of their goals and does not limit their thinking.

How you could do this

Richard Bandler and John Grinder, the founders of neuro-linguistic programming, noticed that, when communicating, people adopt three methods – which they named 'deletion', 'generalisation' and 'distortion'– in the way they use language (Bandler & Grinder, 1975). People use these methods to explain their experiences to others without going into great detail.

We all use these processes every day when communicating. We do this by being selective and *deleting* detail and information when telling our story. We make *generalisations* by transferring the conclusions reached from one experience to another. We *distort* reality by misinterpreting information and/or letting our imagination run riot.

The Meta Model (Bandler & Grinder, 1975) provides some questions to enable us to overcome the deletions, distortions and generalisations that people make. The questions are ones that you might naturally ask when you want to clarify meaning and help someone avoid thinking-traps and obstacles which block their progress.

Deleting

This is the process by which we filter details of experience. When we talk to someone, we economise on what we tell them:

'John is a good person,' (This does not tell us in what way he is good, who to or if there are people he is not good to.)

'I'm afraid.' (Who or what is the person afraid of? Are they afraid of everything or something specific?)

'I don't like him.' (This does not tell us what they do not like about the person, or why.)

Filtering information in this way is helpful in some situations, but creates misunderstanding and can be misleading in other ways because the listener may well fill in the deletions and jump to their own conclusions.

To avoid this you will need to ask questions to help you gain more information or expand the other person's viewpoint. Figure 25 gives some examples.

Deletion-type statements	Questions to gather more information
'I find it easy to make changes.'	*'Which changes have you found easy?'*
'I'm no good at relationships.'	*'What specifically do you find difficult when forming a relationship?'*
'They are out to get me.'	*'Who is out to get you?'*
'I handled the situation badly.'	*'Compared with what or whom?'*
'I have no confidence.'	*'In which situations do you lack confidence?'*

Figure 25 Examples of asking questions to gather more information

Generalisations

Generalisation occurs when we transfer conclusions from one situation to fit other similar situations. It allows us to build on existing knowledge and use the same methods to address different circumstances. However, when we extend a statement or conclusion to cover all possibilities, this can give rise to problems. Consider the following:

'Men are afraid of commitment.'

'Your family will always be there for you.'

'All criminals have troubled backgrounds.'

'Politicians are corrupt.'

'The customer is always right.'

'Rich people are greedy.'

Are these generalised statements always true?

Generalisations can usually be spotted by the use of words and phrases such as 'all', 'every', 'I always', 'I never', 'I must', 'I should', 'I ought' and 'I have to'. Frequently, as in some of the statements above, these are implied.

Rigid, 'black-and-white' thinking does not allow for exceptions about people and situations and closes down any opportunity for looking at other options and possibilities. Listen for these verbal clues to how the person is restricting their thinking and encourage them to take a wider perspective. Do this by asking questions such as:

'What would happen if you did ...?'

'What is stopping you ...?

'Have there been occasions when this didn't happen?'

'What would happen if you could ...?'

'Can you think of a time when you were able to ...?'

It is useful to work with the person to help them replace restricting words and statements such as 'I must ...', 'I always' and 'I have to...' with alternatives such as 'I choose to ...', 'I have decided to ...', 'I want to ...' or 'I like to ...' These statements then acknowledge that there may be alternatives and choices.

Distortions

Distortions happen when we misinterpret incoming information. We might make assumptions about something or presume we know what someone else is thinking without any evidence. Often these assumptions may be based on what we might feel or think in the same situation. For example:

> 'My tutor thinks I'm stupid.'

> 'I know Jane doesn't like me.'

> 'He doesn't look at me when I'm talking. He's not listening.'

> 'I know Peter won't like this.'

> 'He didn't show it but he disapproved.'

The problem with distortion is that it does not always represent the truth. Have you ever watched a film or read a book and had a different understanding from someone else of what it was about? We interpret things in the light of our own experience, which may not be the same for other people.

Creativity depends on the ability to distort reality to make interesting and new connections. Literature and art distort to entertain and amuse us. We also use it to dream about the future we want to make for ourselves. However, creativity is unhelpful when we try to mind-read or make judgements about other people without gathering more information and specific facts.

Questions to ask in these instances include:

'How do you know ...?'

'Can you explain to me how ... means that ...?'

'What leads you to believe ...?'

Comment

The Meta Model provides an excellent way to gather information, clarify what someone means, identify ways in which they are limiting their thinking and help them overcome obstacles. Do be aware, though, that there is danger in gathering too much information. Ask yourself: *'Do I really need to know this to help the person gain their desired outcome?'*

Do keep in mind that asking too many questions, particularly in an abrupt way, can come across as aggressive. Think about ways in which you can turn questions into statements, such as: *'Tell me why you think ...'* or *'Help me understand why ...'*

You might also like to apply some of these questions to yourself, to examine your own use of language. What *deletions*, *generalisations* and *distortions* are you using? How might they affect your relationship with the service user?

SECTION 6

Making positive use of relapses (Relapse)

During the process of change – and of maintaining it – the person may have several relapses: this is normal. These relapses need to be used – to learn from the experience, the person needs to try new, more effective options and to plan to avoid further relapses.

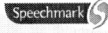

Strategy 40: Examining what triggered relapse

Introduction

Relapse does not usually occur because the person has made a conscious decision to go back to their old habits. They may be lulled into a false sense of security and tell themselves it will be OK to ease up on an exercise programme or expose themselves to situations in which temptation is present. This begins a gradual slide back into old habits. Distress and social pressures are also major causes of relapse into former behaviour. It is essential to examine what triggered relapse and to adjust action plans to take this into account.

How you could do this

People underestimate how much effort is required to achieve change. Often, behaviours are established over a long period of time – frequently many years. It is not realistic to expect to be able to make changes without a great deal of effort, commitment, perseverance and time. It usually takes many months to establish new patterns of behaviour. Often, people are unprepared for complications or are tempted to substitute one problem behaviour for another. They may take a very 'black-and-white' view and feel that if they lose their temper once or give in and, say, have a pudding, that is it – they have failed.

Bear in mind that individuals may not be prepared for their emotional reactions and might deal with them by eating, drinking, smoking, becoming angry, feeling guilty or other irrational thinking and behaviour (see Strategy 31: 'Dealing with emotions'). Social pressure may be another cause of relapse. Individuals may need to make substantial changes to their social networks to avoid being pressured back into old habits. These issues, and others that apply, need to be teased out and addressed.

First, establish at what stage of the change process the person is now. Have they become completely despondent about their ability to make or maintain the change, so that you need to go back to the beginning and arouse their interest again? You may need to remind them that few people succeed in making changes to long-standing problems at a first attempt. It is part of the process of learning from experience. They may be at a stage when they have decided they still want to change and are ready to look again at their action plan and make adjustments to it, to take into account whatever triggered their relapse. The process needs to be picked up at whatever stage the person has gone back to.

Remind the person about Kolb's learning cycle (see Strategy 32: 'Monitoring progress') and how they can use experience in order to learn. They will need to revisit and confirm their decision to change and may even decide to change their goals. Help them identify what led to the relapse and which specific actions they could use in order to deal with similar situations in the future. These will then need to be incorporated into their action plan, or a new plan developed. Be sure to discuss and ensure that they take into account how they will deal with slip-ups and complications so that these do not develop into further full-blown relapses.

When this process has been completed, the person is ready to move on to the action stage and continue the cycle. It is important that the service user is ready for this commitment. If they are not, they may need to do more preparation work in order not to fail again.

Most people will gain from the fact that they have previously taken action. This usually provides additional strength and determination.

Comment

In some environments it is easy to start thinking in a negative way, particularly when other staff have adopted a negative attitude towards a service user and that person is seen as troublesome or difficult, perhaps having had several relapses. You might have thoughts such as: 'This person can't change' and give up on them. Or other staff may make comments which can trigger negative thoughts: 'Is this worth the effort?', 'Wouldn't it be easier to use punitive methods and ban the person from the dining room permanently?' Challenge this self-talk! It will transmit to the service user and have a negative effect on your relationship and their belief in their ability to change. If you do not believe that change is possible for them, how are *they* going to believe it?

 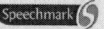

Strategy 41: Reviewing values and beliefs

Introduction

Sometimes values and beliefs which the person initially thought were important (see Strategy 5: 'Establishing values and beliefs') are now less significant and others, which they thought less important, have been shown to have more meaning for the person than first thought. Also, the person may have given some values importance because they represented how they would like to be seen by others, rather than those values having intrinsic significance for them. If someone is trying to act on a plan which is not true to them, this is likely to cause stress, anxiety and lack of real enthusiasm, commitment and motivation. If you have identified that this has been an influence on the person relapsing, it will need to be revisited.

How you could do this

You can either go back to the beginning (see Strategy 5: 'Establishing values and beliefs) or, if you are aware of what the person originally presented as their values and beliefs, look again at these statements. One way to do this is to ask the person to mark how important each original value is to them at the present time on a scale of 0 to 100. They can add any other values they now feel have become important. This can be done on a sheet of paper – for an example, see Figure 26 (overleaf).

You will see from this what has now become most important to the person. Discuss the original plan of action to see whether it aligns with these values and beliefs. Adjustments may need to be made to allow for any disparity. Goals and some actions may need to be changed. Make sure the person retains what worked well and discuss alternatives for actions that no longer align with current values and goals.

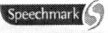

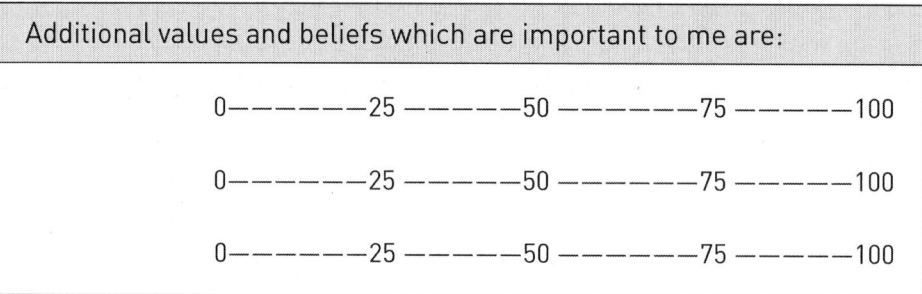

Mark on each scale how important this value or belief is to you.			
Being loyal	0———————25 ———————50 ———————75 ———————100		
Having fun	0———————25 ———————50 ———————75 ———————100		
Having a career	0———————25 ———————50 ———————75 ———————100		

Additional values and beliefs which are important to me are:
0———————25 ———————50 ———————75 ———————100
0———————25 ———————50 ———————75 ———————100
0———————25 ———————50 ———————75 ———————100

Figure 26 Example of values and beliefs scales

Comment

The process discussed above needs to be accomplished using active listening skills and highlighting any disparities in a way that is non-threatening, avoids argument and allows the person to maintain their sense of control. They choose and decide on any changes to the approach. Lead them into adopting an attitude that if one thing does not work, they need to try something else – also, that life is a constant process of change to which we all need to adapt.

Strategy 42: Breaking habit patterns

Introduction

Many people have great difficulty breaking old, unhelpful patterns of behaviour. After a short time they revert to previous behaviour and ways of coping with difficulties or events. This is not surprising. They could have practised and reinforced an old pattern of behaviour or way of coping for many years. These may be habits learned from within the family and passed on through each generation. They might include, for instance, overeating when stressed, reverting to losing one's temper and being abusive when confronted by a problem, feeling overwhelmed or having to acknowledge one is mistaken, closing oneself away, drinking excessively, smoking, or wilfully ignoring that there is a problem.

Trying to break an old habit such as overeating or being aggressive can be a little like becoming stuck in deep ruts formed by other vehicles when you are driving. While you stay in the ruts, steering is easy, but if you try to pull out of the ruts onto firm ground, handling the vehicle becomes difficult. You will have to struggle to avoid being forced back into the ruts. Once on firm ground, you may fall back into them a few times when negotiating difficult obstacles or if you lose focus. There will be feelings of anxiety and discomfort at times during this period. This is completely natural and a period through which the person can be supported – they can be taught some tactics to use to keep them on firmer ground.

How you could do this

First, establish what the unhelpful behaviour pattern is and what has triggered the relapse. This might be unhelpful self-talk, or the person has allowed anger to build up – they felt overconfident and allowed it to happen gradually; or the strategy they were using did not work for them, it was too big a step in one go; or their language patterns (see Strategy 39: 'Understanding what people say') show that they are being selective in their thoughts and deleting positive details in their story – not allowing a more positive stance. They may also have made generalisations or distorted information, with the result that their imagination has run riot and led to the relapse.

Having teased out what triggered the relapse, the next step is to enable the person to plan how this can be dealt with in the future. It is better if they come up with ideas themselves that they feel will work for them but, if they have difficulty doing this, here are a few ideas that you could suggest they consider.

- Break the pattern gradually – one small step at a time. They can try an experiment to see how it feels. Small successes will provide the impetus and confidence to take a further step.

- Remember that they need to make a start on creating a new pattern before they can get rid of an old one. This needs to be a pattern that gives them what they want and can be sustained. If it feels like a punishment, it will not work and will need to be changed.

- If something does not work for them, they accept and acknowledge the fact and do something different that is more likely to succeed. They can ask themselves: *'What is stopping me from trying something different?'* or *'I wonder what it would be like if I tried ...?'*

- Watch out for unhelpful self-talk and language patterns. They can change if they want to and if they have the right support.

- Ask for help and support when they need it. They should be selective and ask the right people. Asking for help from someone who is unable to give it, or who does not have their best interests at heart will not be helpful and can be obstructive.

- Watch out for and weed out beliefs and values that are obsolete, no longer useful or do not contribute to what they want.

- Avoid building mountains to climb. They need to keep things separate. If there is a problem in one area, such as taking part in a group, being in the dining room, doing something in particular, or with a particular, issue, discourage them from saying things like: *'This always happens to me'*, *'Nothing ever works out for me'* or *'I always get things wrong.'* They need to be specific: *'I have a particular problem in groups when ...'*, *'I sometimes get things wrong when ...'* or *'I find it difficult to say "No" to John when he ...'* In this way, the particular issue can be confronted and a solution worked out. It makes a big difference.

- Stop allowing unhelpful responses to problems or difficulties becoming a pattern. If they are blaming others or their situation, they will not be able to learn from the experience, and what starts as a response to a concern will become an unhelpful habit that gradually leads to relapse. If it is becoming a recurring pattern, they need to learn from it by looking at the difficulty and finding a way of dealing with it that enables them to achieve their goals.

- Take into account the impact other people have on them. Look out for how they are being influenced and affected by others. Encourage them to avoid as much contact as possible with people who affect them adversely and to seek out those who are helpful.

Comment

Breaking old habits that do not serve our objectives is not easy. Old patterns are comfortable and give a feeling of control and the safety of familiarity. Watch out for individuals who attempt to rationalise their unhelpful behaviour or habit and try to justify it rather than confront it. It is very easy to allow this to lead into an argument about the matter, which will only help build their resistance. Help them take a more constructive approach by asking something like: *'What do you think will happen if you continue to do this?'*

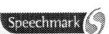

Strategy 43: Trying different approaches

Introduction

The same principle applies to us in whichever role we work – support worker, counsellor, nurse, tutor, mentor – when we are trying to overcome resistance and motivate people. If one approach does not work, we advocate that the service user tries something else. If what we are doing is not working, and the person is not responding, then we also need to try something different: if possible, something that will surprise them.

How you could do this

Acknowledge your role in the person's lack of progress or relapse

This is a technique suggested by Moursund and Kenny (2002). Using this approach, you acknowledge something which you have done or failed to do, or which was inappropriate for the service user, that may have affected their progress or resulted in their relapse. This is intended to lead into an open conversation in which you discuss your relationship with the person, resolve any areas they have concerns about and bring about an improved approach as to how they deal with problems.

The benefits of this approach include:

- Most people blame themselves for their lack of progress or relapse. This approach may relieve them of some of the pressure.

- It may surprise them.

- You are modelling the change and learning process (see Kolb's learning cycle in Strategy 32: 'Monitoring progress'). You reflect on what went well and less well, acknowledge and take responsibility for any errors and areas that could be improved. You also consider what can be learned from the experience, what needs to be changed and done differently, and work towards implementing these changes by seeking feedback from the service user. If you have built good rapport with the person, and it seems appropriate for them, you may decide it would be helpful to discuss the process you have used.

- The person may feel some discomfort that you are taking responsibility for their actions, or lack of them. They may then acknowledge what has gone wrong, take responsibility and be open to discussing their concerns and what needs to change.

Offer a different way of communicating or learning

Most of our communication with service users is done through talking. We assume that they understand everything and that we have understood what they are saying, when in fact this is not so. Service users do not want to appear stupid and unable to find the right words to express themselves in conversation – and think it would be impolite to tell us – and so the process continues, increasing the prospect of demotivation and relapse. In these instances, talking can be combined with the person's preferred communication and learning style, which may include drawing, presenting their thoughts and difficulties in written narrative or poetry, or acting them out in dramatic or even dance form. After talking, writing is probably the most popular method.

Generally, people use a mix of learning styles. Some may have a favourite and make less use of the others. Also, people may make use of different styles in different situations. With this in mind, you can use a mix in the way you present information to individuals, or ask them which they prefer. If they appear to have a favourite, you can lean heavily to that format. You can obtain clues to people's preferred learning styles by listening to the phrases they use. Figure 27 (overleaf) gives some examples.

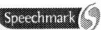

Common phrases	Learning style	How to respond
'I can't see how that would work.' 'I'm having difficulty picturing that.' 'How would I draw that?' 'Do you see what I mean?'	Visual	Use images, pictures, diagrams, colour, mind maps and visual words and phrases
'That sounds OK.' 'I like the sound of that.' 'That rings a bell.' 'I hear what you're saying.'	Auditory	Use recordings, a soft musical background, rhythm and rhyme and poetry, and make aural connections to what you are saying
'Tell me about it.' 'Can we talk about it?' 'I'll spell it out for you.' 'In other words, you're saying ...'	Verbal	Use discussion and writing, record sessions to be played back, speak in a dramatic way using emphasis and avoid using a monotone voice
'That feels right.' 'I can't get to grips with this.' 'No, that doesn't sit right.' 'My gut feeling tells me ...'	Physical	Use role play, practise skills, use touch, action and movement and focus on physical sensations
'That makes sense.' 'I don't see a pattern in that.' 'Can we make a list?' 'That doesn't seem logical to me.'	Logical	Make sure the reasons for what you are doing are clear, highlight logical thoughts and behaviours, present things in a very logical way

Common phrases	Learning style	How to respond
'Can I work with someone on this?' 'Help me understand this.' 'Can we explore my options?' 'Who could I discuss this with?'	Social	Suggest they work with someone, attend a support group, use role plays and share their goals with others
'I need to think about that.' 'Can I come back to you later on that?' 'I think that ...' 'I'll take time out to think that through.'	Solitary	Encourage the use of visualisation, recommend books to use for self-study, encourage them to ask questions to clarify their thinking

Figure 27 Spotting learning styles

Switching how you present information can have a profound effect on your relationship with service users and their motivation. It is something to take into account when examining what triggered relapses.

Discuss what is happening between you and the person right now

This is a way of breaking through barriers and highlighting issues that need to be addressed. This is not something you would normally do in daily conversation and it usually comes as surprise to the person you want to help. To succeed, you need to make yourself consciously aware of what is happening between you, and then state this clearly. The person will feel a bit uncomfortable when you do this, so make sure you approach it in a supportive way and avoid adopting any hint of confrontation in your tone of voice.

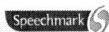

Here are a few suggestions for how this might be achieved:

'John, it feels like I am doing all the work here. You seem distracted. Tell me what is going through your mind at this moment.'

'Lyn, I've noticed that every time we begin to talk about ... you seem uncomfortable and change the subject. It seems automatic. What do you feel when the topic comes up?'

'I sense that something has changed. You seem a bit confused. My attempts to clarify issues seem to make you feel uncomfortable. Tell me what you think might be causing this.'

'Each time we try to talk about your husband's role in supporting you, you flinch and seem uncomfortable. I wonder if you have changed your mind about how he is doing this?'

Using immediacy in this way can help break through the resistance someone has to speaking out concerning what is on their mind. It may also bring to light issues which may have contributed to their relapse.

Put the responsibility firmly in the service user's hands

You can use this tactic when the service user has confirmed their goals, but is reluctant to discuss or deal with the difficulties that have caused the relapse. The idea is to place the issue firmly in the service user's hands and ask them to take responsibility for their own problems. You do this by making a direct statement:

'Tell me how you intend to deal with ...'

'You are clear about your goals, but seem reluctant to discuss your concerns about ... How are you going to overcome that?'

'I sense some reluctance to discuss ... Tell me what would make it easier for you to talk about this.'

Often, the person will say that they do not know. This can mean a number of things, such as:

- You are going too fast for them.

- Not enough rapport and trust has been established.

- You are asking too many questions and it seems like an interrogation.

- You are asking leading questions.

- You are giving advice that is not appropriate.

- The person does not feel in control. Saying *'I don't know'* gives control back to them.

- The person genuinely does not know.

- The answer might be threatening.

- The person has been avoiding facing up to the issue or admitting a fault, feeling that you will not like the answer, or you will think less of them, or they feel ashamed or embarrassed about it.

- They might have an attitude of fighting authority.

- You have shown a bias that opposes making an honest answer.

There are many more reasons that could be in play. Depending on your reading of the situation, there are a number of ways in which you might respond, which could lead into a useful discussion:

'Take your time. At first it can feel really uncomfortable talking about ...'

'You are afraid that if you say what you think I will be offended or take it the wrong way.'

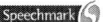

'At the moment you find it difficult to come up with an answer because you are searching for ways to do this.'

'At the moment you don't see any solutions. Would it help if I made a few suggestions?'

'You haven't yet built enough trust in me to disclose this type of information. Perhaps you will feel able to come back to it later when you feel more confident.'

Comment

These are only some examples of different approaches which you may find useful. Discussion with colleagues, staff training and reading will enable you to add to your armoury of resources. You can then apply what is most appropriate in different circumstances.

SECTION 7

Making sure change has been successfully achieved (Permanent exit)

Many professionals believe that the permanent resolution of a problem is impossible. There is always the chance that under pressure of personal disasters or stress, there is a danger of maladaptive behaviour returning. This is probably true for behaviours such as alcohol abuse or weight gain, but with others – such as smoking – it becomes less likely as the person ages. People can, however, be aware of the danger signs and live in a way that avoids the recurrence of self-defeating behaviours.

This entails focusing on maintaining personal responsibility, accepting both negative and positive feelings and being able to recognise and deal with ambivalent feelings.

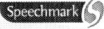

Strategy 44: Accepting negative and positive feelings

Introduction

There are no guarantees that life will go along smoothly and that there will be no high or low periods. Many things in life are unpredictable and we have little control over them. At times of exhilaration, when a person feels everything is going well, they still need to take care that overconfidence does not make them feel they can expose themselves to dangers, such as environments and activities that led to former behaviours. At other times, when there are pressures and difficulties to be overcome and the person is feeling low, warning signs need to be heeded so they do not resort to former maladaptive habits of coping.

How you could do this

When we are aware of, and in control of, our emotions we are able to think clearly, manage stress, be creative, express our feelings and feel confident. When we lose control of our emotions, we can become confused, feel isolated and adopt a negative attitude. We can be tempted to former maladaptive behaviour.

The first step in being able to work through emotional experiences is for the person to acknowledge and accept that there will be ups and downs as time goes on. At varying times, they will feel sad, joyful, angry, bored, anxious, contented, lonely, overwhelmed, motivated and depressed. That is normal. They need to acknowledge and accept that this is the case. They may find it helpful to have a mantra they can repeat to themselves, such as: *'Stop. It's OK to feel bored. Everyone does from time to time. This is normal. I can listen to music. That will help me relax.'*

A good way to help service users become more aware of these changing emotions is to invite them to keep a journal in which they record their emotions on a daily basis for a week or a month. They can do this during a set time every evening, or make a quick note in their journal at different times during the day. They can also note down their thoughts while experiencing the different moods. Doing this will make them aware of their changing emotions and any dangerous self-talk they are experiencing and enable them to challenge and substitute it for self-talk that is more helpful (see Strategy 30: 'Understanding self-talk'). For example: *'It's OK. I'm feeling depressed. I need cheering up. Eating one cream cake won't harm me'* can be substituted with something like: *'Stop! This will get you back into your old eating habits again. You don't want that. If you need cheering up, give Peter a ring.'*

Using the journal, the person can have a range of self-talk options and other actions in place to rein themselves in when they are feeling high, angry or lonely, or to keep motivated when feeling low and to guard against any temptations that could lead into relapse.

Another approach that might suit some is to help the person become aware of danger signs and to recognise that they are becoming vulnerable so that they can take action. For example, a service user might know that when they experience particular emotions, such as becoming sad or depressed, it has been their habit in the past to comfort eat. In this instance, you could work with them to compile a list of signs that indicate that they are becoming depressed. This might include feeling guilty, becoming irritable, withdrawing from or avoiding people, seeing themselves as worthless, seeing the future as hopeless, having difficulty sleeping, losing interest in usual activities, and so on. The desire to comfort eat might also be a warning sign. They then need to decide on what actions they can take to deal with the situation.

A simple form, such as that shown in Figure 28 (overleaf), can be used for this. The person can then keep it as a reminder.

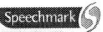

WARNING SIGNS WORKSHEET		
Emotion	**Warning signs**	**Actions I can take are:**

Figure 28 Example of a warning signs worksheet

Comment

It can take a long time to break completely with an old way of coping or an old behaviour so that, regardless of the situation, there is little or no danger of reverting to it. It may take months or years. This is especially so with long- and well-established behaviours and addictions. The temptations may still be there when people are under extreme emotional pressure.

Speechmark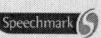

Strategy 45: Encouraging a positive approach to the future

Introduction

An individual's belief in their goals and in their ability to achieve them provides the foundation for motivation and for adopting a positive approach to the future. When events in life are not going to plan, it can be hard to plumb inner resources and maintain a positive attitude. However, service users can be encouraged to take actions which help them sustain a positive outlook.

How you could do this

There is truth in the old adage that the only constant in life is change. This change may be physical or involve health, social life, personal life, circumstances or events over which we have little or no control. Often, previously set goals become obsolete, beliefs which were important become less significant and other beliefs take their place. If the person you are working with is still trying to follow their old goals and beliefs, they may well find themselves becoming demotivated, anxious, bored or dissatisfied and, because what they are doing is out of alignment with their current situation and life changes, they could be tempted back into old habits.

To maintain a positive approach, this process of continuous change – no matter how slow – makes it important for everyone to reflect on their beliefs and goals from time to time, realigning their action plans to ensure they are all in harmony with their life changes (see Strategy 5: 'Establishing values and beliefs, Strategy 23: 'Negotiating goals' and Strategy 24: 'Planning the change'). You can make the service user aware of this, or assist them with it, at regular six-monthly or yearly intervals.

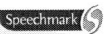

Some other ways in which you could support someone in keeping a positive attitude are by encouraging them to:

- Maintain a support system of people who are rooting for them and have their best interests at heart. These are people who will help them bolster their self-esteem by congratulating them on their successes and reminding them of their strengths: 'You have great determination. I know you can do this', or 'You are really good at organising events.'

- Forgive both themselves and others. Nobody is perfect. Everyone makes mistakes and wrong decisions, or says the wrong thing from time to time. If left to fester, negative feelings of guilt, anger, regret or disappointment can eat away at a person's self-belief and their ability to think in a positive way and get on with life. This can cause all sorts of damage, such as stress, depression or physical illness. Some things which can help individuals learn to forgive themselves include:

  - Remind themselves that what has happened is done. They cannot undo it. If appropriate, they can say that they are sorry or try to make amends if they have hurt someone. If someone has hurt them, they can decide whether they want to face up to that person and deal with it, or let it go.

  - Learn from what happened, so that the negative behaviour is not repeated in the future.

  - Imagine the mistake drifting away into the past and state to themselves: 'I forgive myself (or the other person) for ...'

- Acknowledge and accept positive comments, compliment themselves and stay aware of their own strengths and skills. They can do this by reflecting on comments and confirming them in their mind: 'Yes, I did do a good job. That was a good meal.' They might also reflect on their day and write down the strengths they have shown: 'I was patient and kind with Joan, despite her provocative manner' or 'I made a really good job of the flower arrangements.'

- Focus on what is important. They can do this by spending a short time reviewing their schedule for the past week on a regular basis and calmly asking themselves: *'What did I do that is important to me?'* They can then decide whether they need to cut out any particular activities in the coming weeks and add others of more value that will help them achieve their goals.

- Have a balanced and healthy lifestyle. The areas to keep in balance include:

  - mental well-being: keeping mentally active and ensuring that the person is sufficiently challenged

  - physical well-being: keeping well, physically active and fit

  - eating a healthy diet

  - spiritual well-being: examine from time to time that what the person is doing does not conflict with what they believe or value

  - social life: ensure that the person enjoys a social life and is supported by friends

  - personal life: time for self, personal needs and wants

  - work: is this kept in proportion or does it dominate everything else?

  - finance: does the person lead a lifestyle that is within their means?

- Seek out and associate with people who have similar values, beliefs and goals.

- Ask for help when needed. This might be the support of a 'buddy', a friend or a professional. Anything from a simple chat on the phone to a friend to help from a medical practitioner can be vital in avoiding unhelpful thinking spiralling out of control or depression or anxiety taking hold.

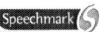

Comment

Keep in mind while discussing these issues with service users that it is best to encourage them to come up with their own suggestions about how they can maintain a positive approach: *'What have you done in the past to stay positive?'*, *'Some people find ... has helped. What do you think?'*, and so on. If ideas are imposed on them, they may feel resistant and are less likely to carry them out.

Strategy 46: Personal responsibility

Introduction

Throughout this book emphasis has been given to placing the responsibility for making changes, and how they go about this, on the service user – *'It's up to you to decide what to do about ... You are the person who will have to do it'* – as advocated by Edwards & Orford (1977). The same principle applies to the service user's future. How the changes are sustained and how they work out is a decision for which they must take responsibility. It is no good for the service user to point a finger of blame at others when things do not go according to plan, or go completely wrong. If they take responsibility and learn to coach themselves through difficult situations, things will quickly improve.

How you could do this

The first priority is to ensure that the service user is in no doubt about who is responsible for them following the path they have chosen. This should be a natural outcome of working with the person. Whether tacitly understood or not, it is best to state this upfront: *'It is your responsibility to ensure that you achieve the life you have decided you want. In order to do this, you may need to use some self-coaching tactics.'* This can be put in many different ways. Some self-coaching tactics, such as using positive self-talk and visualisation, are discussed earlier in this book. Here are some more suggestions you might offer the person.

- **Stay connected to the signposts they have set**. These are the markers or actions they have decided on which tell them how far they have travelled towards their goals. They are usually the answers to questions such as: *'How will I know when I have reached ... stage?'* Stopping at these markers, looking around and congratulating themselves on how far they have come, will help avoid tunnel vision and keep them moving in the right direction.

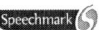

- **Anchor good feelings**. To do this, the person chooses a moment of success and, in their mind, runs through the event several times, noting all the details and how they felt, until they can recall it with ease. When they have done this a number of times, they do it once more and when the experience reaches its highest emotional point, they press their middle finger and thumb together. They can do this a few times. Pressing their finger and thumb together in this way will enable them, in the future, to replay their successful experience at any time they need to feel good and in control.

- **Use a 'stay calm' strategy**. This is good for those moments when the person is feeling panicky or afraid, or if their mind is starting to rush out of control. They repeat the mantra 'calm' or 'hush' several times, either aloud or in their mind. Then they imagine themselves in a calm and relaxing place, such as by a mountain stream, in a garden smelling the flowers, in an art gallery looking at a favourite painting, or walking their dog through a field. This will provide space to calm down sufficiently to enable the mind to bring things back into proportion, start working again and enable appropriate action to be taken. A few attempts are all that is needed to find out whether this works for the person.

- **Be clear about boundaries**. This is not a justification for being rude. However, it does mean that when the person says 'No', they mean it. If necessary, they can listen carefully to any concerns the other person has and repeat what has been said to show they have understood. They can then share their own perspective and check that the other person has understood it. They then move the conversation on.

- **Change viewpoints**. If the service user's mind is spiralling into a negative thinking loop, they may be too close to the situation to get a rational perspective on what is happening. One way to distance themselves and bring things back into proportion, and gain new insights and options, is to look at the situation from a different viewpoint. This might mean asking themselves questions from the perspective of a friend, a colleague, an employer or a relative.

How might they see and deal with the situation? This increases flexibility in thinking. It can also enable the person to imagine how their behaviour may be impacting on someone else.

- **Avoid old solutions that did not work**. It is always easiest to take old routes that feel familiar and comfortable. There is an old adage that if you do what you have always done, you will get what you have always got. Encourage the person to continually look for new solutions that take them away from old unhelpful ones. They can ask themselves questions to help with this, such as: *'Was this successful before? If not, what could I do differently to make it work better? What could I do instead?'*

- **Watch their language**. This is a tactic to keep a person thinking in a positive way and help them find unexpected and better solutions to difficulties. Figure 29 shows some words and phrases that people use to describe both difficulties and other, more helpful, ways to think, which would not only lift their mood but also enable them to think more creatively about solutions.

Common ways to describe situation	More helpful ways to think
'I feel stuck.'	*'I'm looking for a way to move on.'*
'I'm confused.'	*'I need to focus on ...'*
'I have a problem.'	*'I'm trying to find another way to ...'*
'I feel lonely.'	*'This afternoon I could ...'*
'Nothing works.'	*'What could I change or where could I seek advice to make this work?'*
'I can't do this.'	*'I can't do this, yet.'*

Figure 29 Examples of helpful ways to think

To do this, individuals practise and change from stating things as a problem to rephrasing the sentence in a solution-focused way.

Start by asking them to write down, in a daily diary, problem-focused statements they make. They can then spend time rephrasing these in a solution-orientated way. After some practice, they will begin to automatically catch the thoughts as they occur and learn to change them on the spot until, finally, it becomes natural to react in a more helpful way.

Continually challenge their thinking. When they come up against a problem or a block, the two most important questions are: 'What would happen if I could do this?' and 'What would need to happen for me to be able to do this?'

Comment

It is surprising the difference it makes when individuals accept responsibility for themselves and their future. They suddenly become more positive, their mood lifts and their confidence builds. Acquiring self-coaching skills will enable them to maintain that outlook.

REFERENCES

Bandler R & Grinder J (1975) *The Structure of Magic 1: A Book about Language & Therapy*, Science & Behaviour Books, Palo Alto, CA.

Constantine JA, Stone Fish L & Piercy FP (1984) 'A systematic procedure for teaching positive connotation', *Journal of Marital and Family Therapy*, 10 (3), pp313–16.

Dobbie A & Tysinger J (2005) 'Evidence-based strategies that help office-based teachers give effective feedback', *Family Medicine*, 37, pp617–19.

Edelman S (2002) *Change Your Thinking*, 2nd edn, ABC Books, Sydney.

Edwards G & Orford J (1977) 'A plain treatment for alcoholism', *Proceedings of the Royal Society of Medicine*, 70, pp344–8.

Gordon T (1970) *Parent Effectiveness Training*, Wyden, New York.

Kolb D (1984) *Experiential Learning*, Prentice Hall, Englewood Cliffs, NJ.

Lakoff G & Johnson M (1980) *Metaphors We Live By*, University of Chicago Press, Chicago, IL.

Lambert T (1996) *Key Management Solutions: 50 Leading Edge Solutions to Executive Challenges*, FT Pitman Publishing, London.

Luft J (1969) *Of Human Interaction*, National Press Books, Palo Alto, CA.

Maslow AH (1954) *Motivation and Personality*, Harper & Row, New York.

Maslow AH (1971) *The Farther Reaches of Human Nature,* Viking, New York.

Maslow AH & Lowery R (eds) (1999) *Towards a Psychology of Being*, 3rd edn, Wiley, New York.

Miller WR & Rollnick S (1991) *Motivational Interviewing*, Guildford Press, New York.

Moursund J & Kenny MC (2002) *The Process of Counselling and Psychotherapy*, 4th edn, Prentice Hall, New Jersey.

O'Hanlon W & Weiner-Davis M (1989) *In Search of Solutions: A New Direction in Psychotherapy*, WW Norton, New York.

 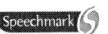

Pearson J (ed) (2011) *Concise Oxford Dictionary* 12th edn, Oxford University Press, Oxford.

Prochaska JO & DiClemente CC (1982) 'Transtheoretical therapy: towards a more integrative model of change', *Psychotherapy: Theory, Research, and Practice*, 19, pp276–88.

Reynolds D (2002) *A Handbook for Constructive Living*, University of Havai'i Press, Honolulu.

Rogers CR (1967) *On Becoming A Person : A Psychotherapist's View of Psychotherapy*, 2nd edn, Constable, London.

Rollnick S, Miller WR & Butler C (2008) *Motivational Interviewing in Health Care: Helping Patients Change Behaviour*, Guildford Press, New York.

Further reading

There are many books available on the various approaches – and many address specific issues. Listed below are a few general books which are fairly accessible and will add to your knowledge.

Motivational interviewing

Dunn C & Rollnick S (2003) *Rapid Reference to Lifestyle and Behaviour Change: Rapid Reference Series*, Elsevier Health Sciences, London.

Prochaska OJ, Norcross JC & DiClemente CC (1994) *Changing for Good*, HarperCollins, New York.

Rollnick S, Mason P & Butler C (1999) *Health Behaviour Change: A Guide for Practitioners*, Churchill-Livingstone, London.

Solution-focused therapy

MacDonald AJ (2007) *Solution-Focused Therapy: Theory, Research & Practice*, Sage, London.

O'Connell B (2002) *Solution Focused Therapy (Brief Therapies Series)*, Sage, London.

Winbolt B (2011) *Solution-Focused Therapy for the Helping Professions*, Jessica Kingsley, London.

Neuro-linguistic programming

Bandler R, Roberti A & Fitzpatrick O (2013) *The Ultimate Introduction to NLP*, HarperCollins, London.

O'Connor J & Seymour J (2002) *Introducing NLP*, HarperElement, London.

Young P (2007) *Understanding NLP Principles & Practice*, Crown House, Carmarthen.

Cognitive behaviour therapy

Kinsella P & Garland A (2008) *Cognitive Behaviour Therapy for Mental Health Workers: A Beginner's Guide*, Routledge, Hove.

Westbrook D, Kennerley H & Kirk J (2011) *An Introduction to Cognitive Behaviour Therapy: Skills and Applications*, Sage, London.

Whitfield G & Davidson A (2007) *Cognitive Therapy Explained*, Radcliffe, Oxford.

 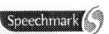

APPENDIX

Guiding principles questionnaire

As you reflect on your work with a service user, ask yourself the questions below and state how you fulfilled each guiding principle.

Guiding principle	How I did this
Have I adopted an empathetic style and used active listening skills?	
Have I been careful with the language I have used?	
Throughout, did I adopt a tone of informing the service user rather than persuading them?	
Did I identify what stage the person is at in the change process?	
Did I help the person clarify the changes they need to make?	
Have the risks of not making the change, as well as the advantages, been fully explored and clarified?	
Have obstacles been identified and removed?	
Did the person confirm desire, ability, reason, need and commitment for the change?	
Did I help the person clarify their goals?	
Did the service user take the lead when setting goals?	

(continued)

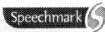

Guiding principle	How I did this
Were alternatives explored so the person could make a choice?	
Were both 'driving' and 'restraining' forces identified that maintain the status quo, and 'driving' forces increased and 'restraining' forces undermined?	
Did I help the person break down their goals into small achievable steps and develop strategies to carry them out?	
Have I given the person clear and frequent feedback about their progress?	
Have I used appropriate communication styles throughout – following, directing and guiding – as required?	